W9-BBZ-450

CHANGE IN THE WEATHER

CHANGE IN THE WEATHER

LIFE AFTER STROKE

MARK McEWEN
with DANIEL PAISNER

GOTHAM
BOOKS

lad 07/09
3

GOTHAM BOOKS
Published by Penguin Group (USA) Inc.
375 Hudson Street, New York, New York 10014, U.S.A.
Penguin Group (Canada), 90 Eglinton Avenue East, Suite 700, Toronto, Ontario M4P 2Y3, Canada
(a division of Pearson Penguin Canada Inc.); Penguin Books Ltd, 80 Strand, London WC2R 0RL,
England; Penguin Ireland, 25 St Stephen's Green, Dublin 2, Ireland (a division of Penguin Books
Ltd); Penguin Group (Australia), 250 Camberwell Road, Camberwell, Victoria 3124, Australia (a
division of Pearson Australia Group Pty Ltd); Penguin Books India Pvt Ltd, 11 Community Centre,
Panchsheel Park, New Delhi—110 017, India; Penguin Group (NZ), 67 Apollo Drive, Rosedale,
North Shore 0632, New Zealand (a division of Pearson New Zealand Ltd); Penguin Books (South
Africa) (Pty) Ltd, 24 Sturdee Avenue, Rosebank, Johannesburg 2196, South Africa

Penguin Books Ltd, Registered Offices: 80 Strand, London WC2R 0RL, England

Published by Gotham Books, a member of Penguin Group (USA) Inc.

First printing, May 2008
10 9 8 7 6 5 4 3 2 1

All photos courtesy of the author, with the exception of the following:
Insert page 2 (center): courtesy of CBS News; page 3 (center right): courtesy of CBS News;
page 4 (center): courtesy of Coca-Cola Company; page 4 (bottom): courtesy of CBS News; page 6
(top center): courtesy of Sabrina Williams; page 8 (top right): courtesy of Sarah Rachel
Photography and Community Services for Adults and Children.

Gotham Books and the skyscraper logo are trademarks of Penguin Group (USA) Inc.

LIBRARY OF CONGRESS CATALOGING-IN-PUBLICATION DATA
McEwen, Mark, 1954–
    Change in the weather: life after stroke / by Mark McEwen with Daniel Paisner.
        p. cm.
    ISBN 978-1-59240-371-4 (hardcover)   1. McEwen, Mark, 1954—Health.   2. Cerebrovascular
disease—Patients—Biography.   3. Cerebrovascular disease—Patients—Rehabilitation.   I. Paisner,
Daniel.   II. Title.
    RC388.5.M284 2008
    362.196'810092—dc22
    [B]   2007049599

Printed in the United States of America
Set in Berkeley
Designed by Ginger Legato

While the author has made every effort to provide accurate telephone numbers and Internet addresses
at the time of publication, neither the publisher nor the author assumes any responsibility for errors, or
for changes that occur after publication. Further, the publisher does not have any control over and does
not assume any responsibility for author or third-party Web sites or their content.

This book is dedicated to Maya, Jenna, Miles, and Griffin
... and especially to Denise, the love of my life

CONTENTS

CONTENTS

You Bet Your Life

used to be a physical therapist. I was a hospital corpsman in the United States Navy. I did my training in Bethesda, Maryland, in 1957, and after that I worked on the PT ward with two other hospital corpsmen—enlisted men like myself. It was exhausting work, but rewarding too, and of course we treated our fair share of stroke patients. Now, this was a long time ago, and there have been certain advances in stroke therapy and treatment over the years, but a lot of what goes on in therapy is the same. What I thought was remarkable back then was the way my stroke patients seemed more traumatized by their situation than some of my other trauma patients. You expect the opposite to be the case, but no, sir. You know, you lose an arm, or a leg, or you're in a fire, or something blew up and you caught some shrapnel…you know what you're dealing with. You know something happened, you know what happened, and you're working on fixing it. There's a context for it, a frame of reference, and you move on.

With stroke, oftentimes, there's no context. There's no frame of reference. Nobody plans for this. You may reach a certain age and think to yourself, Okay, I'm in the area. It's like a minefield. My time is coming. I better watch out. But when you're a young man, like Mark McEwen was a young man, and you wake up in a hospital after you go down with something like this—and you do *go down*, buddy!— all of a sudden there's no context. It just hits you. There's no understanding. Most of all, there's no happiness. Whatever joy you had in your life, whatever spring you had in your step, whatever smile you had on your face, it's just gone. For the time being anyway, gone. I used to see these stroke patients, day after day after day, and there would be this look of wonderment on their faces. They were just baffled. Bewildered, maybe that's the best word for it. What happened to them was just so completely beyond their frame of reference that there was no way for them to get behind it, no way to move on.

Understand, I didn't know any of my patients by name—not at first. And I don't remember any of their names, all these years later. They were brand-new people to me, when they showed up on the unit. But after I worked with them just one time, I felt like I knew them. And then I worked with them a second time, and a third, and I knew them better still. There's a real intimacy between a physical therapist and his patient. Yet, no matter what kind of progress we made during our sessions, no matter what kind of understanding my patients managed to come to on their own, there was still that look of wonderment on their faces. I couldn't wipe it off for trying. It wasn't really a depression, although of course they were all sad. No, it was just pure bewilderment, a look that said, "What are we going to do?" Or, "Will I fully recover?" "Am I going to be my old self?"

I didn't have an answer for that look, but we found that answer in the hard work the doctors laid out for us. We found that answer in the time it took to work these people back to how they were. We had a regimen, a routine. We had a game plan. And it's exhausting; it really is. Not just for the patient, but for the therapist, too. It's emotionally and physically draining, and it just taps you out. Sometimes I went home so emotionally drained at the end of one of my shifts that I wouldn't eat dinner. I just crawled straight into bed, slept the full eight, and then I had a huge breakfast the next morning and came back to do it all over again.

But here's the beautiful thing about the human spirit. No matter how hard I worked, my patients worked harder. No matter how physically drained or spent I was at the end of each session, my patients were even more drained, even more spent. It was all on the line for them, so no matter what I put into it, they put in more. A lot more. And they kept coming back, man. They did. I used to tell them they were like a tired old battleship that's been hit and was listing to the side. That's what I caught myself thinking, when I was working with these patients. But I'll tell you something, just as I told them: They were still seaworthy. You bet your life, they were seaworthy. A little time in the yard, and they were back at it. No question. They could do the work, and make the repairs, and get it back. Not right away, but they could get it back. The will to heal, to conquer, to drive, to crawl, to just take one simple step or to hold a glass of water and bring it to your lips, or to make a simple circle on the tabletop with the palm of your hand... it's a powerful thing, it truly is. And it's a wonderful thing to see.

From time to time, I'd catch a patient cheating on his therapy. By cheating I mean, he wasn't doing his exercises the way he was supposed to do them. By cheating I mean, he was going through the motions, but he was doing a kind of end-around. You'd try to educate the patient about the muscles, about which ones did this and which ones did that, and then you'd ask him to make a certain motion and he would go at it like, SHOOT THE JUICE, BRUCE! He would think, Alright, I'm gonna lift this leg, so let's put everything into this one simple motion. Everything! Seems like a good idea at the time, but it won't take you where you want to go. And that kind of thinking needs muscle education because the patient, calling upon *everything,* makes every muscle tighten.

Here's what I mean: Let's say I want you to lift your arm, and to do so properly you have to work the muscles around your arm from the tip of your shoulder down to the tip of your hand. You're weak, or you can't get your body to respond to a simple command from your brain. Whatever it is, it's just not working, but then somehow you discover that there's a way to lift your arm—only it's the muscles in your neck that are doing the work, instead of the muscles in your shoulder that you're supposed to be working. So you go ahead, and do it that way anyway. You take that *everything* approach, but it doesn't get the job done. It just doesn't. Not over the long haul. It might move your arm or your leg or whatever it is you're trying to move, but you're not getting any benefit from it, because over the long haul what you need to do is exactly what your therapist tells you how to do it. Otherwise, you're just going through the motions. That's what we called cheating. You do the work, but you take those little shortcuts.

I always thought it was the darndest thing, the way these patients would try to cheat on you. You caught them at it and said, "You're not supposed to be doing that." Or, "Is that how your therapist showed you to do it?"

They would just shrug, kinda sheepish, and mumble to themselves. So you'd go at them again.

"Yeah, well, why are you walking like that?"

Again, they would mumble.

"Because you didn't think anybody would know, is that it?"

It's not like riding a bicycle. No, sir. You know that old expression, the one that says once you've learned how to ride a bicycle all you need to do is hop back on and you'll ride again. It doesn't matter if you haven't been on a bicycle in fifty years. You hop back on and you're good to go. But it's not like that with a stroke. It's just not. In fact, this is the one case where that saying just doesn't apply. You don't know how to think, because you have to be re-educated to know what the muscles will do.

So jump ahead fifty years. I get this call from my friend Mark McEwen—this beautiful, wonderful, honest soul of a man you're about to spend some time with in these pages, and he told me what he had been through and it took me back, man. It did. All the way back to that PT unit. Right away, I was a hospital corpsman again, working with my patients, facing down that inability to grasp what was going on. Helping them to deal with their loss of movement, their loss of privacy. It was one big giant *loss,* you know.

There I was, back in that mind-set, thinking about Mark, and the bewilderment I knew he'd faced, the hopelessness, the not knowing what to make of the whole deal. It was all on him, all at once, and my heart broke for him and for his family. It truly did. Not that Mark needs any of us feeling sorry for him, because it's not about that. He has too much fight in him to let it be about that. He has too much want in him to let it be about that.

See, the Mark McEwen I knew was this warm, gentle, funny guy I saw on the television, doing the weather. He had a real way about him. (He's still got it, of course, because stroke can knock you down, but it can't change who you are.) There's something about these weathermen on television that makes you warm up to them right away. I had three of them on this old Groucho Marx game show I used to do, *You Bet Your Life*: Mark, who was on CBS at the time; Willard Scott, from NBC; and Spencer Christian, from ABC. All three network morning show guys. Nicest guys you could hope to meet. Friendly. Cheerful. Quick-witted. The whole package. And they all did an impromptu stand-up routine on our show. We didn't tell them about it beforehand, but we asked them to take the microphone and start riffing for us—and, man, they riffed. Mark most of all. I didn't know this at the time, but he really was a stand-up comedian. A monologist. He had a quick, clever mind, and he did his thing, and he was funny. Man, he had everyone in that studio laughing, and it wasn't any one thing he said or any one joke he told. It was the way he brought you into his world. Like he does here in this book, and that's what I want to get at here. I want to put it out there that the spirit Mark had before his stroke is the same spirit he has now. The stroke couldn't take that from him, and he didn't have to fight to get it back. It was there all along. You can bet your life on that, just as Mark has done, and that's one of the great messages he puts out here. Everyone reading this book, if and when that time comes, or if it's already on you, know that your spirit is intact. Know that if it's a friend or a family member who has been hit by a stroke, that person is still inside.

Yes, it will take time...time...time. And yes, it will take work...work...work. But you'll get there, you will. As long as you don't go looking for any of those shortcuts, you will gain, depending upon the damage. Trust me on this, you will gain. And trust Mark, too, because he's well on his way, also.

—Bill Cosby, 2008

CHANGE IN THE WEATHER

When the world says, "Give up,"
Hope whispers, "Try it one more time."

—author unknown

INTRODUCTION

It Ain't No Use to Sit and Wonder Why, Babe

This is a book about stroke. Specifically, it's about a massive stroke I suffered on Tuesday, November 15, 2005, on a plane home to Orlando, Florida, from Baltimore/Washington International. This massive stroke followed a smaller stroke two days earlier that left me feeling weak and nauseated. Those symptoms drove me to an emergency room visit at a Baltimore-area hospital, where a doctor misdiagnosed me with the stomach flu, sent me home, and told me to get some rest and drink plenty of fluids.

It's also a book about me. People say you should write what you know. I know me, and I know stroke. This strikes me as funny, because up until a couple years ago I didn't know the first thing about stroke. I didn't know the second thing either. To be sure, I knew about me—but you could have barely filled a thimble with what I knew about stroke. Now I travel the country giving speeches to stroke survivors and their caregivers and families. I talk about warning signs and treatment options and aftercare considerations. Mostly I talk about how I survived my own stroke with the support and encouragement of my family and friends and therapists, but before I get to that happy ending I talk about how I naively followed that emergency room doctor's advice and did as I was told. I talk about some of the horror stories I've collected along the way, and how misdiagnosis and misinformation seem to play a role in a lot of stroke cases. It's like the opposite of that old maxim, "What you don't know can't hurt you." With stroke, it's more like, "What you don't know *can* hurt you." Heck, it can kill you. It nearly killed me.

A lot of the folks I talk to recognize me from television. They see someone they invited into their homes over breakfast, or into their bedrooms as they got dressed for work. They remember the long career I enjoyed at CBS News, first as a morning show weatherman and later as an entertainment reporter and eventually as a coanchor. Some of them remember how I spun a pie-in-the-sky, seat-of-the-pants turn as a stand-up comedian into a viable run as a rock 'n' roll radio disc jockey and then into a long-running gig as a network news personality. Of course, they want to hear about my experience with stroke, that's the baseline for our visit, but they want to hear about it from a familiar face. While we're at it, they also want to hear about the unlikely career I managed to build at CBS; the front-row seat it provided to world events like the Olympic Games, political conventions, and Super Bowls; and the lasting friendships it helped me to forge with people like country music superstar Garth Brooks, singing legend Tony Bennett, my boyhood idol, Hall of Fame pitcher Bob Gibson, and President George H. W. Bush. Ironically, it was President Bush who signed the bill designating the month of May as National Stroke Awareness Month, back in 1989, more than fifteen years before I could recognize its importance.

It's all tied together, the life I lived before my stroke and the life I'm living now, and I believe this is an important point. It reminds people that the lives they lived before stroke will come back to them in time, and it reinforces that stroke doesn't discriminate. It doesn't care about race or class or religion. It doesn't care if you've had a long career in morning television or an anonymous career behind the scenes. It cares only about risk factors like high blood pressure and cholesterol and obesity, and whether or not you smoke or drink or exercise regularly.

I'll write more about these risk factors a bit later on in these pages. For now, let me get back to me for a moment, to help set my rehabilitation and recovery in a kind of context. What a lot of people don't remember is that when I worked at CBS I made most of my living in harm's way. For fifteen years, I was the guy the producers asked to do the stunts. Before me, network morning shows featured weathermen, like my good friend Willard Scott, who were known for dressing in silly or outrageous outfits, or for saying silly or outrageous things. After me they had to go out and do stuff. And not just any stuff. It had to be exciting, perilous stuff. At first it just had to be silly or outrageous—to match the outfits and the outbursts, I guess—but then it had to be stuff any rational person wouldn't even consider doing.

By the end of my long tenure at CBS, I was probably the only on-air network news personality with a "reckless endangerment" clause in his contract that actually required him to risk his life. This is a joke, of course, but it's rooted in truth. I should know, because I was the guy they sent parasailing in ripping winds. (I almost drowned when they finally brought me down.) I was the guy they put in the air show plane, or in the race car, or at the top of the Leaning Tower of Pisa for no apparent reason other than it looked a little thrilling and seemed like a good idea. I was the guy who emerged from a coffin to the music of *The Phantom of the Opera* to open our Halloween show one year. I was the guy they put in a barrel in the middle of a bullring in Jackson, Mississippi, while a rodeo clown baited a not-too-happy bull into charging me. (It might as well have been another coffin.) I was the guy who rode the runaway dogsled in Lillehammer, Norway, that careened out of control. I was Walter Mitty, with protective gear.

Yep, that was me.

I was the guy who stood in as the honorary Longhorns

quarterback and took a couple snaps from center for the University of Texas football team. Ricky Williams was a freshman, and on the first play I handed the ball off to him. That was easy enough. On the second play, I hit the wide receiver about fifteen yards downfield with a perfect spiral. Also easy enough.

On the third play, a defensive end named Chris Atkins broke through the line and hit me so hard I thought I saw birds and stars, like in the cartoons. Harry Smith and Paula Zahn were our anchors at the time. They were in an auditorium on campus, where we had set up a remote studio as part of our tour of the state of Texas. They were watching me on the monitors, along with a studio audience comprising mostly Longhorn fans. They all saw me get hit. I was miked, so they all heard me say, "Oooof!" very loud. This, apparently, is what you say, very loud, when you get hit by a three-hundred-pound defensive lineman. "Oooof!" It's not really a word. It's not even an exclamation. It's just the sound you make when all the air leaves your lungs in a painful instant.

This got me on *Entertainment Tonight*, only not in a good way. It ran as a kind of blooper. They showed the footage of Chris Atkins tackling me. They played the audio of all that air leaving my lungs. Then they showed all the other players jumping on top of me, which I guess was meant to show what a rollicking good time they were all having at my expense. After that, they showed my colleagues in the studio, laughing it up. And finally they showed me, crawling my way out from under the pile and staggering to the camera. I took off my helmet and said, "I have a daughter!"

Man, I couldn't believe that quarterbacks get hit that hard a dozen times a game, and still get up and get back out there. I was sore for a week. I tried to laugh it off, but it hurt. I left the field telling Chris I would sue him after he went pro, when he had some real money.

Yep, that was me.

I was up for almost anything, an aspect of headstrong character that would serve me well as I recovered from stroke, although occasionally I took some convincing. Once, in 1992, at the XVI Winter Olympics in Albertville, France, my producer Kevin Coffey spent a week getting me to agree to be buried in six feet of snow so viewers at home could watch an avalanche dog try to sniff me out. Kevin and I had worked together for years. He's one of my closest friends. He knew my thresholds for pain and indignity and danger, and I knew his penchant for ratings and "good television" and the kinds of remote stunts that got our viewers talking, so it was an intense negotiation. He wanted what he wanted, which was to get me to do something outrageous, while I wanted what I wanted, which was to return home from Albertville in one piece. Kevin tried to tell me that it would be a public service, for me to submit to his avalanche dog stunt, to get people to be more careful in the mountains, but I wasn't buying it. I just thought he wanted to bury me in the snow for the cameras. On the first Monday we were in France, he came up to me and asked if I'd agree to it.

I said, "No way."

On Tuesday, Kevin pitched the idea to me again. He said, "How would you like to be buried in the snow?" It was as if we never had that first conversation. He reminded me that these avalanche dogs made life-and-death rescues, and that highlighting these rescue efforts might be helpful to people in avalanche or whiteout situations.

I said, "No way."

On Wednesday, he came at me again.

Once again I said, "No way." Only this time Kevin must have heard something in my voice that made him think I was softening. I was tired of saying no, but I wasn't softening. I had no interest in being buried in all that snow, in creating a life-or-death situation for myself that might not turn out to the good.

By the time Kevin approached me on Thursday, he'd worn me down. We'd worked together much too long by this point; he knew how to manipulate me. Plus, he made it sound like no big deal, like I'd be covered in just six inches of snow. So I finally agreed, and on Friday I showed up at our remote location in the Albertville countryside, not really knowing what to expect. For one thing, when we left the Olympic Village in the valley, I didn't even know what kind of snow we'd find up in the mountains, if we'd find any snow at all. The lack of snow was a constant topic of conversation in the Olympic Village. When we first got to Albertville, the streets were bare. I thought, Maybe we have the wrong Olympics. I was a big fan of the Summer Olympics, so I thought I could adapt. But I quickly learned that in Albertville they clean the streets so fast they don't even give the snow a chance to accumulate. Up in the mountains, in the countryside, there was plenty of snow. The biggest snowflakes I had ever seen were falling all around. There was so much snow that avalanches were a big problem, which was why they needed dogs like the one I was about to meet. Every winter, we learned, there were dozens of hikers and climbers and skiers caught in avalanches, so it was important for us to call attention to the good work done by these dogs and other rescue agencies.

I arrived at our location, and Kevin showed me the hole they had dug for me. It wasn't just a hole. It was more like a grave. Six feet in the ground, and big enough for a guy like me to lie down comfortably and say good-bye to all my worldly concerns. I said to Kevin, "You expect me to get in there?"

He nodded.

I said, "No way."

He said, "It's already set up. The dog is here. You can't back out now."

I said, "But it's a grave."

He said, "No, it's just a hole."

Paula Zahn was with Harry Smith at our studio. She could see the whole setup on the monitors. She could hear the back-and-forth between me and Kevin. She said, "You're going to put Mark in there?"

She said it like a challenge, like she didn't think I could handle it or survive it. There was always a good-natured rapport between me and the anchors, and here it sounded like Paula was egging me on. So what could I do? I got in the hole, and as soon as I did, some guys in the crew started shoveling snow on top of me. They worked quickly, like they thought I might change my mind. Let me tell you, it's eerie and weird and more than a little unsettling to climb into a grave and have a bunch of guys start to bury you with shovelfuls of snow. Luckily, the snow was light and fluffy, but what I learned was that even light and fluffy snow can get heavy and not-so-fluffy when you pile six feet of it on top of you. Someone dug a little cavity for me, so I could breathe. Another someone walked me through what was about to happen. I could even see a little bit, because somehow the daylight was able to penetrate through the snow. I wouldn't be able to breathe for very long, but I could breathe for a while. And I couldn't really see anything but shapes and shadows. I could hear what was going on above me on the surface, though. I was miked and wired, so they could hear me and I could hear them.

When it came time for the segment, the dog's handler held a piece of my clothing to the dog's snout and instructed him to start searching for me. I listened to what was happening through my headset. The dog had been trained like a bloodhound. The catch was that he'd be working through six feet of snow. The handler didn't point this particular dog in any particular direction, although if the dog had been smart he would have been watching just a few moments earlier when they started to bury me. He would have looked up from his hair and makeup chair, or wherever it was they were keeping him while the humans prepared the scene, and started taking notes. But the dog wasn't that smart. He was just a good avalanche dog. He started sniffing, and moving about in circles. His circles got smaller and smaller, each time around, until the dog got very excited when he reached the patch of snow above where I lay. He started digging. He barked as he dug. He kicked up so much light and fluffy snow it looked like he had a snowblower at his feet. Finally, he dug down to where I was, only he was so excited he didn't stop digging or barking. He almost took a bite out of my face, he was so excited. I was plainly terrified. I was thrilled to have been found, and dug from my fluffy-white grave, but at the same time I was scared out of my mind, to look up and find this beast bearing down on me.

Yep, that was me, too. For fifteen years, that was me. Putting myself in harm's way because my producers thought it would make for good television. Taking one for the morning news team. Rising to meet every challenge, no matter how reckless or foolhardy it might have seemed at the time. And I never complained. I might have resisted, but I never complained. I might have been terrified, but I never complained. And then one day, two years after leaving the network for the slower, safer pace of local news, I was once again in harm's way, only this time I hadn't put myself there. This time, harm's way found me. And this time I'd be fighting for more than just ratings. This time I'd be fighting for my life.

All of which takes me in a backdoor sort of way to the series of strokes I suffered in November 2005, because in the end this is a book about how stroke can pull you from the people you love and the plans you've made and the things you enjoy and the career you've built. It's about how stroke changes everything, and how it can leave you wondering if there was anything you might have done differently to prevent it. It's about how stroke can pull you from what you know and love, and how it can return you to these things and instill a new and profound appreciation for them. That's how it happened for me. Every relationship I had was suddenly more resonant, more meaningful. Every sweet moment was now bittersweet as well. More than that, everything I knew, everything I was, everything I believed was now open to reinterpretation. Time and rehab might help me to regain all my faculties and erase almost every deficit left behind by my stroke, but I would be forever changed, just as the people closest to me would be changed by their proximity to my ordeal.

I've had a charmed life, make no mistake about that. I've gotten to do things most people only dream about, and I'm raising four beautiful children with a woman I spent my entire adult life believing I was destined to marry. I was, and remain, deeply and truly blessed, and I know it in my bones that I'm lucky to be alive. But I didn't think these things at the time, when I was first facing the reality of stroke. I do now, though, and this is a book about all this, too. It's a book about all the "Why me?" questions you ask yourself, when you're suddenly felled by a random act of illness. I was a good person. I lived a good life. I helped little old ladies across the street, and I was straightforward. I even took reasonably good care of myself, although I probably could have exercised a little bit more and eaten a little bit less. And still, these strokes managed to find me. You can take care of yourself all you want, I realized. You can be as good and bighearted as they come. You can take as many foolish risks as you want to for fifteen years in front of a television camera and get away with all of them. The bad stuff can still find you.

Why me? I asked myself that question a bunch of times, and I never came up with a good answer. The good news here is that I no longer ask the question. With time and perspective, it no longer seems so important. *That*, friends, is what this book is about. It's about how we move on, how we manage the unmanageable, how we get past the rough patches.

Read on and see if some of the lessons I've learned about life and stroke and rehab might help in your own circumstance. I certainly hope so.

EVENT

What a Long, Strange Trip It's Been

I t started with a road trip.

I went home to Maryland to see my best friend, Tony Colter, and my little brother, Chris. My wife, Denise, said I should go. She thought it would be good for me to have some time for myself. She likes her time, and she likes me to have my time, and here she thought I needed it. I'd been working at WKMG in Orlando for about a year, anchoring the local morning and noon newscasts, and the hours were catching up to me. Awake every day at 3:00 A.M. for the morning news. Asleep every night by 7:30 P.M. I liked being a local news anchor, but the schedule was tough. Unrelenting. My body clock was upside down and inside out. *Jeopardy* was my *Tonight Show*.

It gets to you, after a while. A road trip seemed like just the thing, so I kissed Denise and the kids as I tiptoed out of the house early Friday for my predawn commute, did the morning and noon newscast at WKMG, and headed out for the airport. I'd packed my bags the night before. It was the second week of November, 2005, and I had a busy weekend planned. The night before I left, apropos of nothing, Denise asked me if I had ever been in the hospital overnight. I told her I once had arthroscopic surgery on my knee, but it was only an outpatient procedure, and that was it for me and hospitals. I don't know how the conversation started. We were just talking, and I mentioned how I'd hardly ever been sick. It never occurred to either one of us that my experience with hospitals was about to change.

Maryland is home, so visits there can get complicated. I actually didn't tell my sister or my father that I was coming in to town, because I didn't think I'd have time to see everybody. I didn't want to rush through one visit just to get to another. That's one of the things I'll always regret, because of what happened. It reminded me that it doesn't matter how complicated things get, there's always time for family, even if it's just a rushed visit. Nothing is more important. Even a quick hug is worth squeezing in.

My brother picked me up at Baltimore/Washington International—BWI to us locals. He had an appearance that night at a club. He's a radio deejay, just like I used to be. Baltimore was where I got my start, at WKTK-FM. It was a good place to begin. In radio, the deal is you have to start out in smaller markets and work your way up, so Baltimore was just right. It was already halfway up the ladder, in terms of market size and exposure and salary, and far enough from the top that I could learn on the job without jeopardizing my career prospects. I took home about $100 per week to start, with the added bonus that I could live at home and my friends and family could listen in. I'd had a hard time convincing my parents that I was going to make something of myself, but here they could tune me in on their car radio and check on my progress. They could *hear* I was amounting to something.

My brother had taken a different approach to his radio career. Baltimore wasn't a stepping-stone for him the way it had been for me. He'd decided to make his life and career there, and he was doing great. He's got the same McEwen voice, the same sense of humor, the same passion for rock 'n' roll. He's eleven years younger than me, so he's like a new and improved Mark McEwen. His professional name is Kirk McEwen. He came up with that name when he was nineteen. There was another deejay on his station then with same first name, Christopher, and they told him he'd have to change his name. The other guy was there first, so I guess he had squatter's rights. It took me a while to get used to calling him Kirk. I liked his real name better. Whenever I went on his show, he had to remind me not to call him Chris on the air. It would be bad for his image, he said, and it might confuse his audience. So I called him the Kirkster instead. His wife, Kelleigh, never knew him as Christopher.

She only knew him as Kirk. He'll probably kill me for putting his real name in this book, but he's my baby brother. I don't care what they call him on the radio, he'll always be Chrissy to me.

We had a nice night. I stayed at my brother's house. I saw his three-year-old daughter Tatum, my goddaughter. It wasn't too often that we got to spend time together without my own kids around as well, so I remember it as a special visit. We goofed around with Tatum for a while, then we had dinner, and then we went out to Chris's appearance. I loved watching him do his thing. He had a great rapport with his audience. I was so proud of him, so happy for him. He seemed to love what he was doing—and he was a real natural at it, too. It was past my bedtime but I didn't care. We were having a good time and I was watching my kid brother in his element. After the appearance, we went back to Chris's house and called it a night. I slept late on Saturday morning—late for me, anyway. I don't think I got up until after 9:00 A.M. I felt fine, well-rested, ready to take on the day. I didn't know it, of course, but this was the last morning I'd wake up all pumped and ready to greet the day for the next while.

Chris drove me to Tony's house, which was kind of a big deal. Chris lived in Hunt Valley, just north of Baltimore. Tony lived in Crofton, outside Annapolis. It's about a forty-five–minute drive. I didn't like putting Chris out, but he didn't mind. It gave us some extra time together. Plus, he'd get to see Tony at the other end. Tony and I have been friends forever. Tony's also a deejay, these days on XM Radio, so us radio guys have to stick together.

The first thing Tony and I did after Chris headed back home was take care of a small family obligation. I needed to see my mother-in-law and her sister, Denise's aunt, who was dying of cancer. Aunt Jean—or AJ, as everyone called her. Denise was always crazy about her. This wasn't really an obligation, because I loved Denise's family. I'd known her mom since we were kids. I called her Peggy. Her sister AJ was in pretty bad shape, and I really wanted to see her while she was still able to enjoy the visit. Tony spent some time with Peggy while I visited with AJ. We were at AJ's house, where she was under hospice care. We stayed for a couple hours. We talked about Denise and the kids. We talked about my new job. We talked about being sick and how it can pull you from the things you love.

We talked about the time AJ came to New York and brought me Maryland crabs, which were quite the delicacy. She knew that one way to my heart was through my stomach. She remembered that day. In fact, her son Jimmy brought over crabs for us to eat during our visit, and I have a distinct memory of sitting with AJ that afternoon, eating crabs, enjoying the day, reminiscing and thinking how the bad stuff like cancer never seemed to happen to me. It might hit the people I loved, but not me. I marveled at AJ's quiet strength and dignity, but I didn't think to wonder how I'd hold up under such life-threatening circumstances because that kind of thing was so far from my experience. It never occurred to me that the tables might be quickly or easily turned, and that I'd soon be the one on the receiving end of one of these visits. Why would I think along those lines? Physically, I was feeling great. Strong. Vital. I'd never been gravely ill in my life, and there was no sense worrying about it now.

After a while, we drove back to Tony's house. We stayed in that night. I wasn't tired or anything, and this wasn't any kind of harbinger of things to come, it's just that there was no reason to go out and chase a good time when there was a good time right in front of us. Tony and his wife, Doreen, fixed us a fantastic dinner. I don't think I was too much help, but I was a good guest—I stayed out of the way and reached for seconds and helped with the dishes. We stayed up late, talking. I felt just fine, and it was good to be with old friends, away from the grind of the local news, away from the din of our busy household. It had been a complicated couple days, but it was the good kind of complicated. It had been an emotional visit with Denise's Aunt Jean, but it was the good kind of emotional.

It was turning out to be a restful weekend after all.

Peaceful.

Necessary.

Denise had been right that I needed to get away.

The next day we lounged around Tony's house until it was time for me to head back to the airport. Tony and I played cribbage. For thirty years, we'd been playing cribbage. For those of you who don't know, cribbage is a classic card game, where the points are tallied by pegs. The game is one of the great, common threads running through our relationship. Wherever we were, whatever we were doing, there was always a deck of cards and a cribbage board nearby. We sat around and played and talked. We talked about my new job. We talked about Tony's job. We talked about music. We talked about our kids. Tony's daughter Karley was also my goddaughter, and now she was already in college, so there was a lot to talk about. Thirty years is a long time. The afternoon passed, and soon it was time for me to catch my plane, so Tony drove me back to BWI and dropped me off at the Departures curb out front.

I started to feel strange as I stood in line to board the plane. I'd already been through security, and through the usual paces they now put you through before boarding, and suddenly I felt a little unsteady on my feet, a little woozy. I thought it was no big thing—and yet it was alarming. I called Denise while I stood there on line. She suggested I eat something, and if you know me at all you'll know I'm not the kind of guy you have to say this to more than once. If you tell me to eat, I'll eat. There was still some time before final boarding, so I ate. Anyway, I meant to. I found a pizza place and ordered a slice. It was airport pizza—not the most appetizing meal for a born-again New Yorker who had grown used to the best pizza in the world, but it didn't look half bad.

The woman at the pizza place was a little rude. It was the strangest encounter, and I wonder now if maybe the woman was acting strange because I was acting strange. Maybe she was bored, at the tail end of a long shift. Or maybe I was putting out some kind of bad mojo, and she was just putting it right back on me. Whatever the reason, the pizza lady wouldn't give me the slice until I paid the money, and I remember thinking it was an unusual way to sell pizza, but then when we finally completed the transaction I didn't feel like eating. It's not like I had any appetite to begin with, but now I didn't even have the motivation to eat. I just wasn't interested in food. This wasn't like me at all, but I didn't really give it a thought.

The next thing I knew, I was signaling to an airline employee at the gate that I needed some help. I said, "I think something's wrong." I can still hear myself getting out these words. My voice sounded like it belonged to someone else, like I was underwater. For some reason, I remember worrying how to tell these airline people what I was feeling, how to get the help I needed, and this was what came out: "I think something's wrong."

There, I thought. That should do it.

I couldn't shake thinking that my future health and well-being was somehow tied to how I managed to communicate what I was feeling to these perfect strangers. This was more than a little unsettling, because at just that moment I had no idea what I was feeling. I couldn't put it into words. There was something "off," that's all. I needed help. And soon it was on its way.

Airline personnel called for an ambulance. By this point

I was having difficulty standing. I can't imagine what I must have looked like, or the scene I was undoubtedly making. I'd always thought of myself as an okay-looking guy, but here I'm sure I looked horrible. Here I'm sure I looked like one of those people you see coming and hope doesn't sit down next to you. Someone walked me to a chair and helped me to sit down and waited with me for the EMT guys to arrive. I don't think I waited too long. I called Tony while I was waiting and told him what was happening. I told him I wasn't going to make my plane, and that I was probably going to go to the hospital. I thought I sounded calm and matter-of-fact, but Tony must have picked up the alarm in my voice, because he said he would come back and meet me and that I should call him as soon as I knew which hospital they were going to take me to. Then I called Denise again and told her what was happening. She was worried, but she wasn't too worried because I tried not to sound too worried. I told her I thought it was probably some type of bug. It could have been something I ate, only I hadn't really eaten anything. Hopefully, whatever it was, it would just be a twenty-four-hour thing. Denise agreed that it was probably nothing serious, and that it was probably a good idea to stay in Maryland another day. Certainly, I was in no shape to fly.

Tony met me in the triage area of the emergency room. I was drifting in and out. Tony told me later that I threw up a lot. I suppose I did. I don't know what I was throwing up, because like I said I hadn't really eaten anything, but I was heaving just the same. If you've ever had the dry heaves, you'll know it's not the most pleasant experience. The room wasn't spinning, but it might as well have been. I was pretty dizzy, pretty nauseated. Tony stayed with me the whole time. A doctor came in and out. A nurse came in and out. There were all kinds of people looking in on me. Not a single one of them uttered the word *stroke* or gave any indication that what I was suffering was anything serious. Someone mentioned my high blood pressure, which they thought might be relevant. I'd been diagnosed with high blood pressure, and was taking medication for it. When I was first diagnosed, I told people I just had "a touch" of high blood pressure, but then I met a doctor who told me it's either high or it's not. It's like being a little bit pregnant. Anyway, everyone I knew in television news seemed to have high blood pressure. It seemed to be an occupational hazard. But, relevant or not, my condition didn't seem to concern the doctor assigned to my case, and so it didn't concern me. What did I know about health and medicine? What did I know about stroke? What did I know, even, about high blood pressure? All I knew was that I went to the hospital in an ambulance and a bunch of doctors and nurses and people in white coats checked me out pretty thoroughly. Everyone seemed serious and professional and good at their jobs. Everyone seemed genuinely, but not overly, concerned. I still felt miserable now that they were done checking me out, but the consensus was that I was merely suffering from a case of stomach flu, so after being at the hospital for just a couple hours they sent me home. If anyone had even hinted that I might have suffered a stroke, I wouldn't have been so quick to leave, but a stroke was the furthest thing from my mind because it was also the furthest thing from everybody else's mind.

Tony drove me back to his place and I holed away in his guest bedroom, hoping the sickness would soon pass. As soon as we got back to Tony's house, I called Skip Valet, the WKMG news director. Skip was my boss. I needed to tell him I wouldn't be able to do the news the following morning. This wasn't an easy phone call to make, in part because I didn't feel like talking but also because I knew what it meant to the station if I missed a newscast. It was November, which in the world of television meant it was a sweeps month. This was the time of year when our ratings mattered most of all, because it determined our advertising rates for the rest of the year. Skip was a good guy. We'd only known each other a year or so, but already I considered him a good and trusted friend. He told me to take whatever time I needed, but in his voice I heard, *Hurry back*. After all, this was why he'd hired me, to boost ratings, so to disappear during sweeps was a big deal.

We talked briefly, and for the first time that day I thought about stroke. I thought about it because Skip brought it up. He brought it up because one of our colleagues at the station had recently suffered a stroke while she was on the air. Her name was Cecily Wilson, and she was WKMG's on-air traffic reporter. She was delivering her segment one morning and started slurring her speech. She dropped a bunch of words. It was a disquieting thing. Frightening, too, only none of us really knew enough to be frightened at the time. I'd never seen anything like it before, and I didn't know what to make of it. I instructed the director to turn the camera on me and picked up Cecily's report and tried to cover for her. The first thing I thought was that I hoped she didn't embarrass herself. It's not the most compassionate first thing I could have thought on Cecily's behalf, but I didn't know anything about stroke, about the damage it could cause, so I only thought about the damage it might do to her career. Skip knew right away that Cecily was having a stroke. As it turned out, happily, Cecily suffered only a mild stroke. In fact, it was so mild she was able to drive herself to the hospital immediately afterward. She was in the hospital for about a week, and returned to work soon after, and now you can listen to her give one of her reports and have no idea she's had a stroke. Now she's as good as new.

I remembered, of course, but it wasn't a front-and-center memory. I hadn't made the connection to what I was experiencing. Why would I make any connection? No medical person had mentioned stroke. Nobody else had mentioned stroke. I'd never really spoken to Cecily about what she was feeling at the time, what her symptoms might have been. This was just me and my boss, fumbling for a diagnosis, thinking out loud. I mentioned the conversation later to Denise on the phone, and we dismissed it, because stroke was just not on our radar. It was something that happened to older people, to people with a family history, to people who were not quite as robust and healthy as yours truly. No, this was most likely a bug and it would soon pass. That's what all the doctors and nurses said, and all those doctors and nurses couldn't be wrong.

I was feeling punk. That's what we used to say when we were kids, which basically means I was wiped out. Weak. I didn't sleep much that night, but I had stopped throwing up, so I was just laying there. Still aching. Still without much of an appetite. I lay around Tony's house the whole next day, too. He went to work and left me alone for a few hours. I didn't feel like eating. I didn't feel like moving. I didn't feel like doing much of anything. I did manage to stumble to Tony's computer and make a cursory search of the Internet for information on stroke. That conversation with Skip had got me thinking. I bounced around from site to site, looking to see if my symptoms might fit. I found one site that said stroke was the third-leading cause of death in the United States, after heart disease and cancer. I didn't know that. I found another site that talked about the telltale warning signs of stroke. It mentioned facial numbness, a rapid decline in arm strength, and problems with speech, such as slurring. I didn't know that either. It also talked about how important it was to get treatment at the first sign of trouble.

The reason I remember the warning signs is that they were all bunched together under the acronym FAST. *Face. Arm. Speech. Time.* That's one of the big campaigns of the

National Stroke Association, the Think FAST campaign, which tries to get people to pay early attention to symptoms. But I couldn't recognize myself in these symptoms. My face wasn't numb. I could lift my arms just fine. My speech wasn't slurred. At least I didn't think my speech was slurred at the time, although some months later, when I was talking over my symptoms with Denise, she corrected me on this. She said a couple of words seemed slurred to her over the phone. She said I sounded a little drunk. Maybe that explained the little bit of weirdness in that exchange with the lady at the airport pizza counter. Maybe I did sound a little out of it, even though in my head I sounded the same way I always sounded.

After a while, I logged off Tony's computer and went back to bed. I slept, off and on. Mostly I just lay there. When Tony came back from work, we played some more cribbage. He thought it would help me to relax, and to take my mind off how I was feeling. He was right. It did. But only a little.

By Tuesday I thought I was ready to get on a plane. I was anxious to get home, and back to work. I spoke to Skip that morning, and he was thrilled when I told him I might be able to do the Wednesday morning newscast. That might have been wishful thinking on my part, and I realize now that recovery is all about wishful thinking. It's about setting goals and heading out to meet them. But I wasn't really thinking about goals, or willing myself back to good health. All I was thinking, really, was that I wanted to sleep in my own bed and get back to my own routines.

I was feeling a little better, a little stronger, but just as a precaution I called ahead to the airline and arranged to have an attendant meet me at the curbside check-in with a wheelchair. This was Denise's idea, and it was a good one. I don't think I would have thought of it myself, and even if I did, I don't think I would have done anything about it. I was too proud to be pushed around the airport in a wheelchair, too self-conscious. But Denise encouraged me to put aside my pride and take every precaution, so I also made arrangements for a wheelchair on arrival in Orlando. Denise didn't say anything, but she knew that if I was so quick to agree to her idea about a wheelchair something must be wrong. As for me, I didn't think something was terribly wrong, just wrong enough to justify the wheelchair. I told myself I could avoid the hustle and hassle of racing through these airports, so for this reason alone it was a good move. And it was, although I must admit I felt a little uncomfortable, being whisked around the airport. That was for the old folks, I thought, or folks with disabilities. Me, I was just a road-weary guy feeling a little punk. What was I doing in a wheelchair?

At one point, when I was sitting by the food court, I noticed an elderly woman crossing to get herself a soda, so I got up from my wheelchair and walked to the counter to get it for her. I don't know why I did this. Maybe I was being chivalrous. Maybe it was just out of habit. Maybe I wanted to show anyone who happened to be looking on that I wasn't some pathetic old coot in a wheelchair. Probably I just wanted to convince myself that I was fine, but by the time I got back to my wheelchair I was spent. That's what I was doing in a wheelchair, I guess. I couldn't have made it through that big terminal on my own steam. No way. I couldn't even cross the food court without needing to sit back down.

I walked onto the plane with the pre-boarders. Looking back, I think I must have grabbed onto the seat backs a little too tightly as I made my way to my seat. I was a little wobbly on my feet, and needed the extra support. There was no one else in my row when I sat down, but I was soon joined by an attractive woman who sat next to me. She wanted to talk. I wanted to sleep—or, at least, to stare blankly through my window and try not to throw up. It was my seatmate's first trip to Orlando. She was concerned about the humidity. I smiled and told her it wasn't the humidity she had to worry about, it was the heat, which of course was an odd piece of insight from a former weatherman, but she seemed to take in stride. After a while, the talk trailed off, and I don't remember too much about the flight after that. I might have slept, but I don't think so. Mostly I just zoned out. The flight attendants didn't pay much attention to me, as I recall. If I could have curled up in a tight ball and disappeared, I would have surely done so, but as it was I could only wait out the rest of the flight.

When the plane started its descent, I suddenly found I couldn't talk. I tried to say something to the woman sitting next to me, to ask her if she too was experiencing the same strange sensation, but no words would come. I couldn't even think where to start, to make myself understood. I tried to move, to reposition myself in my seat to get more comfortable, but my muscles wouldn't respond. It was as if I was paralyzed, and it was a terrifying realization, but then the terror left me as quickly as it had appeared. Then I just closed my eyes and hoped I was having a bad dream, but when I opened them I saw it was no dream. I was right there in my seat, confused and disoriented and unable to move or even communicate. I was there and not there, all at once. I learned later that I was experiencing a massive stroke, compounded by the stroke I'd experienced two days earlier, but of course I couldn't know any of this at the time. I could barely tell you my own name.

I have one clear memory of our descent. I was trying to make sense of a senseless thing, this sudden sickness and weakness and paralysis, when I looked out the window and saw the sun looming over the horizon. It struck me just then as the most beautiful sight I had ever seen. There I was, unable to move a muscle without tremendous effort or even to speak, and alongside this agony was this picture of sheer beauty and wonder. Really, I was fairly lucid and coherent, and it was one of those bizarre freeze-frame moments that pass over you with a thousand tiny story lines attached to it, and you have a thousand different possibilities to consider about what it might mean, and another thousand to consider once you run through the first batch. Probably it just lasted a second or two, until I zoned out all over again, but it's stayed with me. It's like a picture postcard I carry, commemorating my descent into months of rehabilitation and recovery. I close my eyes and see that beautiful skyscape, a backdrop that gave no clue to the stroke that was trying to kill me.

That's the thing about stroke. It's like a stealth missile. It sneaks up on you, often without warning, sometimes right in the middle of a joyful or beautiful moment. Even if you see it coming, you don't know what it is. You don't know to get out of the way.

A flight attendant actually had to shake me alert when the plane landed and people started to get off. I wasn't asleep or passed out, but I was out of it just the same. I remember trying to reorient myself, and then trying to stand up and not doing a very good job of it. My balance was off. I reached for the seat backs again, for support. I had to be helped off the plane. I was a mess—and, a handful.

Somehow, I made it off the plane and into the wheelchair that was waiting for me at the gate. A skycap wheeled me through the airport. This was a little more upsetting than it was at BWI, because here in Orlando, if you looked hard enough, you could find my mug on a couple WKMG ads. Let me tell you, that's an unnerving thing, to be so out of it that you need wheelchair assistance and at the same time you're being wheeled past these giant billboards with your picture on them. The effect was a little too surreal. It doesn't happen this way for most people, I don't think. A part of me thought folks were looking at me like they knew who I was, but I was too out of it to make any eye contact with anyone.

I could not have made small talk if my life depended on it, which was kind of ironic because my life did depend just then on my ability to communicate what I was feeling.

To someone.

Anyone.

On the way to the main terminal, I tried to call Denise on my cell phone. I was aware of recognizing the need to call her, and making the effort to do just that, but at the same time I don't think I was fully aware of what I was doing. I managed to press the speed dial for home, but I couldn't bring the phone to my ear or say anything into the mouthpiece. All I could do was speed-dial. I did this six or seven times, although Denise remembers it as more like nine or ten times. (I'll go with her estimate on this.) She told me later she was a little freaked out, to see my number show up on the caller ID nine or ten times like that, over and over, without anyone talking. At first she thought I couldn't get a clear signal, and that it was just a glitch in the technology, but ten times is a long time without a clear signal. She knew me well enough to know that if I didn't have service I would have probably set the phone aside until service became available. But for some reason I kept calling, so of course she became concerned. She connected this concern to the symptoms I experienced at the airport in Baltimore and knew something was horribly wrong. I could hear her say, "Hello," but I couldn't answer. I couldn't talk, but she could hear me breathing. On the fifth or sixth call, she was able to pick out the sounds of the airport. At the

Orlando airport, there's one of those shuttle trams that goes from the gates to the main terminal. There are prerecorded announcements that tell you when and how to board the shuttle, and other by-now familiar messages, so Denise finally heard these announcements in the background and began to piece together where I was and what was happening. She could hear it wasn't a weak signal. She just couldn't hear me.

On the next-to-last call I managed to bring the phone to my ear and to mumble the words, "Help me. Not good." Once again, I think it came out sounding like I was underwater.

Meanwhile, Denise and I had still not really spoken. You'd think the skycap might have noticed I was in distress, and struggling to make a call on my cell phone, but he didn't. He had a package to deliver—namely, me—and he could not see or consider anything else, so he guided me off the shuttle tram toward the exit. Let me tell you, this was one focused skycap. Nothing could distract him from his job, not even the fact that he was wheeling a disoriented guy through the airport who couldn't seem to manage such a simple thing as placing a phone call. When we finally got outside, the skycap left me alone by the curb. My carry-on bag was resting on my lap, where it had been placed by one of the flight attendants when I sat down in the wheelchair. I didn't really notice it at the time, or think anything of it, but I couldn't have said anything or moved to stop him if I did. The clueless skycap had to have seen I was in bad shape, but I guess he thought his job was done. He'd delivered me to the curb, after all, and now all I could do was sit there with my bag in my lap, my hands fumbling with my cell phone, my condition worsening by the minute. I could have died there, and this skycap never would have thought he'd done anything wrong.

Before I worked in radio, I struggled for a time as a stand-up comic. I had an act. I used to perform at places like Catch a Rising Star, in New York and Los Angeles. I look back now and think, something like this, me trying to raise my wife on the phone while a skycap wheeled me around the airport, could have yielded a good couple minutes of material. It was such an absurdly comic scene. You have to laugh about it, I think, otherwise it's just too painful and frustrating and maddening.

Poor Denise was about to lose her mind on the other end of the phone. I speed-dialed her again, and this time I could hear she was frantic with worry. I could hear her screaming, "Hand the phone to someone! Hand the phone to someone!" By this point, she must have put two and two together and figured out I was unable to speak. Certainly, she could tell I was in distress. She said, "Hand the phone to someone who can call an ambulance!"

An overweight gentleman standing to my left seemed to prick up his ears. He was smoking a cigarette. We made eye contact. I tried to flash him a pleading look, and to indicate the phone, which I had fisted clumsily against my face. He could see I was having a hard time. He moved toward me and pointed to the phone. He said, "Do you want me to take that?"

I nodded.

He ended up saving my life, this overweight guy with the cigarette who just happened to be standing on the curb outside the Baggage Claim area having a smoke. He talked to Denise for a moment, then he used my phone to dial 911. He made the call, and answered a few questions for me, and then he left before I even had a chance to thank him. He just handed me back my phone, snuffed out his cigarette, and went back inside to Baggage Claim.

Meanwhile, Denise was frantically trying to track me down from our kitchen phone. We lived in Seminole County, and the Orlando airport was located in Orange County, so when Denise called the Seminole dispatcher she at first had some difficulty getting information on the call that had been made from my cell phone in Orange County. To make things even more confusing, the airport had its own 911 response system, so Denise had to retrace the call yet again. She'd never called 911 before, and here she had to navigate her way through three different emergency dispatch systems before finding out where I was and who had taken my call. It was a whole other absurd comedy of errors. It just went on and on, until Denise was finally put through to the airport 911 dispatcher and was told that there had indeed been a call made by a man matching my description, and that I could now be seen on an airport camera sitting in a wheelchair and talking to paramedics. Denise had no idea if this was a welcome piece of information or another frustration, because of course she thought I was completely unable to speak. She told me later that she thought, Okay, this paramedic is talking to my husband, but my husband couldn't have been saying anything in response. She didn't think anything good could come out of such an exchange, and yet there was nothing she could do from the phone in our kitchen except to wait for the situation to play out on its own.

The ambulance took me to Sand Lake Hospital, which I just assumed was the closest hospital to the airport. I couldn't speak, but I was clearheaded enough to know that this was how it worked, that they have to take you to the nearest facility and not necessarily the best facility for whatever treatment you might need. As it turned out, Sand Lake was probably the best place for me, but it was just dumb luck that I wound up there. I can still remember the EMT guy who rode with me in the back, telling me I was in good hands. It was a reassuring thing to hear. He told me not to worry, so I tried not to worry.

Denise met me in the emergency room at the hospital. I hoped someone had been reassuring her, telling her not to worry. I was alert, and happy to see her, and trying to put the best face on the situation. We talked for a moment. She asked how I was feeling. I said, "Not so good. How do I look?"

She laughed.

I remember the nurse who checked me in. She took my

temperature, my pulse, my blood pressure. She said, "When did you first notice something was wrong?"

I said, "A couple days ago."

The nurse frowned. This was not a good answer, apparently, when you're talking about the onset of stroke—which, also apparently, was what we were now talking about. Here at Sand Lake, stroke was the first thing on their minds in the emergency room. Up in Baltimore, it hadn't been on their minds at all. The nurse flashed a look of concern and said, "That's a long time."

Indeed it was. I later learned that there's a window of about three hours, starting when you first notice the signs of stroke, for a patient to take some proactive measures and either stop the stroke or mitigate its damage. One of the things you can do, depending on the type and severity of the stroke, is administer blood-thinning "clot-busting" drugs that can help minimize the damage of most strokes. In some cases, there are oxygen therapies that are called for to help with recovery. And in still other cases, with a "progressing" stroke such as mine that continues to attack the brain over a prolonged period, you can at the very least be kept under observation until your body stabilizes. If you wait longer than those three hours without doing anything, there's no telling what the stroke might do. Here I'd waited way longer than three hours, and on top of that I'd been unlucky enough to have been on an airplane for the massive stroke, so this nurse must have thought the worst.

I looked over at Denise and saw that she was not laughing anymore. I didn't have a diagnosis or a prognosis or any *osis* other than my usual neurosis, but just from the expression on Denise's face and this nurse's face, I could tell that this was serious.

After that, I don't remember much of anything.

LIFE BEFORE STROKE: *STAND-UP*

My father, Alfred, was a colonel in the Air Force. We lived in places like San Antonio, Texas, and Montgomery, Alabama. We even lived in Berlin. Actually, we logged two separate stints in Germany. The first time, we lived in a town called Zweibrücken. That's where my kid sister Karen was born. After that, we moved to Texas, and then to Berlin. We were in Berlin at the same time as President Kennedy, when he made his famous *Ich bin ein Berliner* speech. I was nine years old. There were police barricades and a tremendous crush of people lining the streets. A guy I didn't know helped me get to the front of the crowd. He said, "You should see your president."

We lived in Berlin from 1962 to 1965. I can still picture it. I even remember the Berlin Wall. I remember finding out we were moving back to the States, this time to a place called Maryland. I had to look it up on a map. This was the final stop for my dad, who retired from the Air Force in 1971 and went to work for the Civil Rights Commission and later for the Library of Congress. My mom, Dolores, worked for Citizens National Bank, first as a receptionist and later as a manager, eventually becoming a vice president.

Maryland is where I place myself when I dream about my childhood. My dad's still there, in the same house in Crownsville where I did the tail end of my growing up. My mom passed away in 2000, but most of the McEwen clan has stayed local. There were six of us McEwen kids. My brother Billy was the oldest. Then came my sister Leslie, then me, then my younger sister Karen and my younger brothers Sean and Chris. It was a busy household, wherever our household happened to be.

Crownsville, Maryland, was where I figured out what I wanted to do with my life. Or, at least, what I didn't want to do. I was a process-of-elimination kind of guy. I didn't want to sit behind a desk or punch the same clock as everyone else. My heroes were comedians and ball players. By the end of high school, I'd ruled out a career as an athlete, so that left stand-up as my only realistic career goal.

I went to the University of Maryland to study people. I went for three and a half years. As a fallback, I worked at the campus radio station, WMUC-FM, as a disc jockey. Radio wasn't necessarily something I wanted to do for a living, but it was a whole lot of fun. I lived for rock 'n' roll, but I also listened to Stevie Wonder, Aretha Franklin, Al Green, and Earth, Wind & Fire. Joni Mitchell, too. I was all over the dial.

By the middle of senior year, I wanted to be a stand-up comedian. I wanted to go to New York. My grandmother lived in Queens, so I thought I knew the city, although in truth I only knew a small part of Queens. But back in the 1970s, New York was like Mecca for stand-ups, so I hopped the next bus to New York, grabbed a room at a YMCA on West 34th Street. I wasn't fool enough to leave school for good on just a whim and an open mike. That would come later. For now, I was only a little foolish. The YMCA was a depressing place. Every time I watch *Taxi Driver*, I can smell the disinfectant they used to clean the floors of that Y. It's one of those smells, it gets in your nose and it ties in to every sense-memory you have about the place. I can close my eyes and picture myself back in that dingy room. I was like Robert De Niro, alone in a cheap boardinghouse, but with jokes.

Open-mike night at Catch a Rising Star was on a Monday. I went up to New York on a Friday. School was still in session. I had it all worked out in my head. I'd take in the scene, and get a feel for the city and the club. Then I'd take the stage, and leave to resounding applause and laughter. I'd be an overnight sensation. Then I'd call down to Maryland and send for my things. There'd be no reason to finish school, once I killed onstage. I'd be on Carson the following week, if everything went according to plan.

I stood outside of Catch with all the other people who thought they could do stand-up, waiting my turn. Richard Belzer was the emcee. He told me I was up next. I went outside to get some air and clear my head. Then I started to walk around the block. I never went back to the club. I walked back to the Y and packed my bag. I was back in school on Tuesday. I'd only missed a day of classes. That's all it took for me to realize I wasn't ready to chase my dream. Or maybe it was that my dream wasn't fully formed. I was overwhelmed that first time on my own in the city. Everything was just out of reach. People had always told me I was funny, but I'd never performed. I'd never gotten up at a frat party or in a coffeehouse and told a single joke. I didn't know you were supposed to write out your material.

My favorite comedians at the time were Bill Cosby and Richard Pryor. I liked Cosby because he was clean and smart. He was also an idol of mine. He could pull a laugh out of any situation. I liked Pryor because he was different and because he totally changed the art of doing stand-up. He'd say anything to get you to laugh, or to think about something in a new way. Me, I was like-able. I had that going for me. People said if you were likeable onstage, that was half the climb. It was the rest of the hill that had me worried.

The second time I came to New York, I was smart enough to watch the comics for a couple nights before I went on. I rented a loft apartment I couldn't afford, I guess on the theory that it would give me a sense of urgency. I wanted to feel like I was living in New York instead of just visiting. There would be more at stake. Also, this time I was foolish enough to leave school, probably on the same sense of urgency. I probably thought there would be more at stake if I didn't have school and the radio station to fall back on.

I watched Rodney Dangerfield perform that first night back in New York. It was like a workshop for him—and a master class for me. Rodney had jokes written on the back of an envelope. If he read a line and it got a laugh, he said, "That's a keeper." If it bombed, he crossed it out and moved to the next joke. I went to the club the next night and saw some of the same comics I'd seen the night before. They told the same jokes all over again. They told them the same way, with the same pauses, the same facial expressions to punctuate the laugh lines. I thought, That's cheating. I also thought, Maybe I should write something down.

I fell for one of the waitresses. It was love at first sight—for me, anyway. I don't think the waitress even noticed me. I finally struck up a conversation with her, and she didn't seem too impressed that I was going on-stage. I guessed in her line of work you met a lot of aspiring comics. It wasn't necessarily a good thing to be, in her estimation. I said, "Just wait 'til you see me up there." I said, "I'm gonna kill."

She said, "We'll see."

I thought, Thanks for the encouragement.

I went out and did my five minutes. I don't think I killed, but I maimed. I said, "Comedy is all about timing." Then I looked at my watch and shrugged and said, "At about two o'clock this afternoon, I was funny as shit." It got a big laugh. I wrote that joke on the way from the bar to the stage.

I never went back to school. I was just a couple months shy of graduation, but I didn't see the point. My father couldn't believe it. He wasn't angry, just incredulous. My parents couldn't understand how a rational young adult could put three and a half years into a four-year program and pull out just short of the finish line. It made no sense to them. But it made sense to me. Going back to school just for the sake of going back to school was irrational, although I didn't stay in New York very long. Eventually, I made my way to Hollywood. That's where you went if you wanted to be discovered. There was a West Coast version of Catch a Rising Star, which was managed by Mitzi Shore, who would later become better known as the mother of Pauly Shore. The

LA Catch was in Westwood, near UCLA. It was more laid-back than the New York Catch, but the comics were just as desperate to get noticed. I did my "comedy is about timing" joke, and it got a laugh. Then I looked at my watch again and said, "It's a little after eleven. We have another twenty minutes to kill until Carson." That got a laugh, too.

After my first open mike performance, Mitzi Shore came up to me and said I didn't have to try out anymore. She said I had what it took to be one of her regulars. She offered me $10 a show. I thought, This was why I left school, to become a regular performer at Catch a Rising Star, for $10 a show? The pay was like dirt, but the money wasn't the only problem with the gig. For one thing, I had to write ten minutes of new material, because regulars were expected to do a ten or fifteen minute set. I thought, How am I going to come up with ten minutes of new material? For another thing, Mitzi had other regulars who were more regular than me. I would go on at two or three in the morning. There was no chance of me getting seen by anyone in a position to help my career, and there was only a slightly better chance of me getting any laughs. Anyone sitting in a comedy club at three in the morning was either drunk or waiting to go on next.

I quickly learned that stand-up comics keep their day jobs. Sometimes, they even add a second. I learned this after trying to stretch my $10 fee to cover my room and a couple jars of peanut butter for sustenance. I worked for a while as a furniture mover. I was a big guy, and I could move stuff, so I was qualified. I had a bunch of different jobs. I was also qualified to be a bank teller. My mom used to hire me to work summers as a teller at her bank, so I went to an employment agency to look for a bank teller job. I had three shirts, and three ties, which added to my qualifications.

I met someone who told me about a youth hostel in Beverly Hills where I could get a cheap room. I thought, Beverly Hills? Even a youth hostel in Beverly Hills had to be out of my price range. Sure enough, there was a room I could afford. It was on Beverly Boulevard. I paid by the week. There was a shower down the hall. And I starved, starved, starved. I'm only now able to look at peanut butter again, because that's all I could afford.

I was twenty-one years old, and I wasn't just broke. I was flat broke. I was also lonely. I missed my younger brother, Chris. This surprised me. Chris was only ten. I don't know why I missed him more than anyone else in my family, but it was probably because he was so young, so innocent. He had his whole life in front of him, and the rest of his growing up to do. I hated that I wasn't around for him, and I hated that even though I had the whole rest of my life in front of me it still felt like I had stalled. Here I was, doing what I wanted, but I was losing hope that I'd ever make a real living at it.

This was where radio came back into the picture. I'd always been a rock 'n' roll kind of guy. I'd always listened to music and talked about music and idolized my favorite musicians. I figured I could parlay my experience at WMUC into an on-air job at some station, somewhere. I took the bus one day to a radio station in Westwood. I had one audition tape, which the guy asked me to leave behind. I said, "When can I get the tape back?" He must have thought, Who is this kid? But it was my only copy. Nobody told me you needed to make copies of your audition tape. I figured it out, though. I made some copies of my audition tape and started sending them around to program directors. Then I sat down and made myself a peanut butter sandwich and hoped I'd catch a break.

SAND LAKE

When You're Weary, Feeling Small

woke up in the hospital two days later. It didn't take long for me to realize that something was terribly wrong and that for the time being at least I was almost completely disabled, although it would be some time before I could put all the pieces in place and get the full picture. It would be six months before I even learned I had been in a coma.

The neurosurgeon assigned to my case suggested to my wife, Denise, that she contact my next of kin, which she did. When I woke up, I looked around my hospital room and thought, This is not good. The room was filled with next of kin, which is normally the best kind of kin, only not when they've apparently gathered to say good-bye. Then they're like a receiving line headed in the wrong direction. I closed my eyes and pictured a morbid version of that scene in *The Wizard of Oz*, when Dorothy wakes from her dream to find everyone she knows in her bedroom, worried sick over her because she had been hit on the head.

Here I was, with a hit to the head of my own, an injury to my brain, slowly gaining consciousness while my father, my sisters, my brother, my best friend, my cousin, my bosses, and my wife came into view. At first I thought, How nice, everyone came down to see me. And then I thought, Oh, no. It's odd, in times of stress, how the brain pieces together what's going on. It might take an extra beat or two, but you figure things out before long, because even an injured brain can put two and two together and not like the answer.

There was a blood clot in my cerebellum, I heard someone say. I'd had a massive stroke, I heard another someone say. I had something called basilar artery thrombosis, I heard a doctor say. I was lucky to be alive. This was the first time I heard that phrase in relation to me, and I would hear it a lot in the weeks and months ahead. It took some getting used to. It may have been true, but at the time I didn't feel all that lucky. I couldn't walk or swallow. I could hardly speak. I could hardly move. *Lucky* was probably one of the last words I'd have chosen to describe my circumstance. Quietly, my doctors worried if I would ever regain these abilities. Also quietly, my wife worried how she'd manage our two small boys and our two older daughters without me around to help out. She worried if I would ever be able to go back to work, if our health insurance would cover my medical costs, if she would have to take care of me for the rest of my life. This was how her brain puzzled together what our future might look like, how two and two added up for her. She went to sleep at night not knowing if I would ever again be the man she married.

Still, I looked around my room and saw almost everyone I cared about, almost everyone who cared about me. Most of them had flown in from out of town. Most of them had already been there for over twenty-four hours. And most of them wore a look that was somewhere between happy to see me and worried sick.

That's a strange scene to wake up to, I'll give you that. When you come to and see all these people, your first thought isn't, Oh my God, I must be in bad shape. Your first thought is, Gee, I'm glad to see everyone. Or, It's so nice of them to take time from their busy lives to come to the hospital to see me. That's as far as it went with me at first. I just thought everyone had come down to see me because they loved me and I was in the hospital, or maybe because there was a family reunion I'd forgotten about, not because I was so close to death. But then I realized that most of them had come a terribly long way, so I started to think, Okay, if they're all here, looking all concerned like that, I must be in deep doo-doo. I hadn't spoken to a doctor yet, but that was my professional opinion, just from reading everyone's expression in the room. I didn't have the presence of mind to think things through any further just yet.

Everything was clear and unclear, all at once. I was in trouble, that's all I knew. I tried to speak, but nothing came out. I had so many questions bouncing around inside my head, and no way to ask them. I had no idea I'd suffered a stroke. I had no idea I'd been in and out of a coma. I had no idea two days had passed since I had to be helped off that plane and rushed to the hospital. At first I thought it was still Tuesday, possibly much later in the day to account for everyone's arrival at my bedside, and then when the calendar didn't quite match up with the passage of time I just figured I'd been disoriented and out of it for a couple days.

During those couple days, my neurosurgeon saved my life. I didn't know this at the time, but there's no overstating Dr. Max Medary's role in my recovery. What a godsend this guy turned out to be. I don't think he was in the room when I first opened my eyes, but someone sent for him double-quick—and it was a good thing, too, because Dr. Medary had some new and aggressive ideas on treating patients with stroke. He wasn't the neurologist on duty when I came in to the emergency room, but he caught my case the next day. Dr. Medary's chief objective was to destroy the blood clot that remained in my cerebellum. He'd described the situation for Denise, who laid it out for me when I came to.

According to Dr. Medary, my stroke was still progressing. I'd never heard that term before, in connection to stroke—but then, I hadn't registered too much in connection to stroke, so what the heck did I know? The stroke wasn't finished with me, was how he put it. The big concern was this clot, which they discovered in my cerebellum when they did a brain scan. It was a big worry, this clot. It wasn't moving, or shrinking, or doing anything at all really. It was just sitting there, threatening my life, because it could have hemorrhaged at any time, or moved in the wrong direction. I never knew a clot could cause so much trouble. A lot of doctors would have left it alone and hoped it didn't hemorrhage, but Dr. Medary thought we should rachet up my blood pressure to encourage the blood flow in my brain and push the clot into submission. It was a dangerous procedure, he explained, because the increased blood flow could also cause me to hemorrhage, but he presented it as our best option.

Dr. Medary was well-known in his field, and he was certainly one of the leading neurosurgeons in Central Florida, but Denise hadn't known enough to seek him out. There was no time to seek anyone out. We didn't know what I was facing just yet, so for the time being we were just going with the flow. The thing I liked best about Dr. Medary was that he was a straight shooter. He was a glass half-empty kind of guy. He told it like it was, without sugarcoating.

I don't think Denise appreciated this approach as much as I did. When she first consulted with him, while I was still out of it, she asked him directly, "He's going to live, right?"

Dr. Medary thought about this for a moment and said, "I'm sorry, Mrs. McEwen, but I can't tell you that just yet."

Then he laid out my situation for Denise in terms she could understand, and explained how increasing the blood pressure was my best chance to survive, and the best way to attack the blood clot. He said that the same treatment that could save me could also kill me, but it was still our best option.

I can't imagine what that must have been like for poor Denise, to have been placed in that kind of dilemma. She must have felt so alone, so terrified. There were friends and family all around, but no one could really help her with a decision like this, and I hate that I was so out of it that this had to fall on her. But she was tough. She was diligent. She asked all the right questions—like, what could happen if boosting my blood pressure turned out to be a bad strategy? (The answer: I could have another stroke, and this one might kill me or leave me paralyzed or far worse off than I was at just that moment.) She reached for the right second opinions. And, when I was finally able to join in the discussion, she shared her view.

As soon as I regained consciousness and was strong and focused enough for a consult, Dr. Medary laid out the situation for me as well. He told me I was lucky—there was that word again!—but that I wasn't in the clear. There was still this clot we had to worry about, and it was a big worry. Unfortunately, my worries didn't end there. Even my best-case scenarios weren't looking all that good, according to Dr. Medary. He told me I might regain some of my physical abilities that now appeared lost, but there were no guarantees. He said we wouldn't know for a while. In any case, he told me I was in for a long, hard struggle, and that I was now more than twice as likely to suffer another debilitating stroke than folks who had never experienced a first. This last was a difficult thing to hear. Surprising, too. I thought, a thing like this, it knocks you down, you should at least get some kind of free pass the next time around, but that's not how it works. It's like once it knows where to find you, it comes back looking for more.

Stroke, I was reminded, is the third leading cause of death in the United States, behind cancer and heart disease. It's also the leading cause of disability among American adults. I'd learned all of this that afternoon on Tony's computer, when I was scouring the Internet for something to explain my strange symptoms, but it was a whole other puzzle knowing that these facts now applied to me. These would be the new facts of my life going forward, stat lines I would come to repeat in speeches and interviews as I traveled the country, telling my story and promoting stroke awareness. The numbers are alarming, and enlightening, and yet at that moment stroke was completely outside of our shared experience so Denise and I were flying blind. I'd known a few people over the years who had suffered a stroke, but I never knew the details or understood what it meant. Was it an injury? An illness? An attack of some kind, like a heart attack? Were there things you could do to prevent it? To ensure your recovery? I couldn't say, but as I regained consciousness at Sand Lake Hospital, I thought stroke was something that only happened to old people—specifically to old people who were frail and in poor health to begin with. Man, was I wrong about that. Stroke can hit you at any time, for any reason—or, for no reason at all. Old or young, fat or thin, family history or no family history...stroke doesn't care. Yes, it's an injury. Yes, it's an illness. Yes, it's like an attack or arrest of your normal brain functions. And yes, there were things you could do to reduce your risk factors and improve your chances of recovery. I would learn all of these things in time, but all I could do just then was try to reconcile my relatively young age, fifty-one, and apparent good health alongside the diagnosis I'd just been given.

Denise was in the same place in her thinking, but Dr. Medary cleared some of that up for us. He also scared us. He'd already scared Denise with his line about how the treatment that could save me might also kill me, and now he was scaring me. I don't scare easy, and Denise doesn't either, but this was tough. Nine times out of ten, Dr. Medary said, patients don't survive the kind of massive stroke I'd suffered. To complicate matters, I'd also suffered another stroke, at the airport that Sunday as I went to take my scheduled flight home. Dr. Medary said I was that tenth guy, the one who survives, but that it would be a while before we knew the full effects of this "event" going forward. That's what they call it, when they're not completely sure what to call it. Stroke, heart attack, seizure...whatever it is, before they make a conclusive diagnosis, they call it an event. They make it sound like the Super Bowl, or a black-tie gala. At this point, Dr. Medary was certain that I had suffered a major and prolonged stroke on that flight home to Orlando.

I closed my eyes and thought, Gee, thanks for inviting me.

I was alive, but I was far from whole. One of the first things I noticed about my condition was that my right hand and leg were essentially frozen—not frozen to the touch, but frozen stiff, like I could fight my way through the thaw if only I worked at it hard enough. That's how it goes with stroke. You feel as if you should be able to will yourself to move, but your body won't respond. And it's typically a one-sided deal. Of course, no one stroke is like another and everybody's brain responds differently to injury, but stroke mainly hits the dominant side of your body, so I couldn't use my right hand. I couldn't lift my right leg. I couldn't raise my right arm. I was fortunate in that the right side of my face was unaffected. A lot of times, you see stroke victims with a pronounced droop on the side of their face where their body suffered the damage, but I didn't get that. I just looked like I usually looked—a little worse for wear, obviously, but essentially the same.

The left side of my body wasn't so great either, but it was in tip-top shape compared to the difficulties I was experiencing on my right side. And it wasn't just that my limbs felt heavy, or that I was too weak to move. It was as if my brain wasn't able to tell my body what it wanted me to do. I could send all the right messages, but they couldn't get through. It took a while for me to process this because I'd always been something of an athlete. I was active, and strong. My body had never failed me before, and here it was failing me spectacularly.

In a huge way.

All of a sudden.

It was a lot to take in. I could understand a good deal of what was going on around me, although a good deal more was muddled. I could follow the conversation, even as I could not actively participate in it. I could pay close attention and connect the symptoms I'd experienced in Maryland to the diagnosis I was now hearing from Dr. Medary. I could even recognize that if my first stroke had been diagnosed in that Maryland emergency room, or even suspected, there was medication I could have taken that would have reduced the risk of subsequent stroke and very likely prevented the second stroke that hit me on the plane. Someone would have noticed that blood clot, and done something about it. At the very least, I would have been admitted to the hospital and prevented from flying.

My brain was working perfectly, in terms of processing information; where it wasn't working had to do with disseminating that information to my voluntary muscles. I could listen in as Denise explained to me what had happened and brought me up to speed. She reminded me how the ambulance picked me up at the Orlando airport, outside the Baggage Claim area, and how she met me here in the Sand Lake emergency room. She told me how she got her ex-husband, my stepdaughter Jenna's dad, to look after our twin boys, so she could stay at my side. She told me how my family and friends raced to be with her and me because the doctors said I might not make it. She left out the part about how I'd been in and out of a coma for the previous two days, and how Dr. Medary suggested she start calling my next of kin, I guess because she thought it might upset me, but she was straightforward about everything else, and I remember thinking what a good job she was doing, taking charge, taking care. Usually, I was the one in our relationship who took charge. Usually, I took care of Denise and our family, but here she was managing just fine.

She has always been my rock, and she would be the family's rock in the days and weeks and months ahead.

Perhaps this is a good spot to tell how Denise and I met and finally got together. I'd known her since she was in high school. The first time I saw her she was cutting grass at her house in Crofton, Maryland. She was wearing a purple tube top. I was drawn to her immediately. Who knows what she saw in me, but apparently she was drawn to me as well. We lived in Crownsville, a couple towns over. Denise was in a driver's ed class with my sister Karen. They were best friends. They're still best friends. Karen thought we should meet, so she drove me over one day on some pretense or other. Denise and I hit it off right away, but we weren't exactly boyfriend and girlfriend. We were together, and not together. Our lives were running on different tracks. She was in high school. I was in college. There was an undeniable connection, to be sure, but at the same time there was a tug and pull taking us in opposite directions.

I remember thinking Denise was like this special gift, only it took years for me to figure it out. I thought we were fated to be together, but consigned to being apart. I learned many years later that she felt the same way. We went around and around with each other, for the longest while. Either Denise was in another relationship, or I was in another relationship. She was living in one part of the country, and I was living in another. Our timing wasn't great, but underneath our lousy timing was a kind of safe haven. We kept returning to each other, in one way or another. In the back of my mind, I always knew we'd wind up together. I think if you ask Denise, she'd say the same thing. There was just a lot of other stuff we had to slog through first, like a couple marriages and career missteps and on and on. Along the way, Denise had a daughter, and I had a daughter, but we still kept in touch.

That undeniable connection never went away.

And now here we were, all these years later, together at last, slogging through a serious set of circumstances neither one of us could have anticipated. Most people don't really pay attention to that *for better or worse* line you hear in most marriage ceremonies, but it didn't get much worse than this. I couldn't really move. I couldn't really talk. I did a lot of listening, as I recall. I also did a lot of nodding subtly, to indicate agreement. The reason I nodded subtly was because anything more forceful was too much of an effort.

Subtly was all I could manage—and even that was a struggle. For some reason, I'm reminded now of that old Faces' album—*A Nod Is as Good as a Wink...to a Blind Horse.* I would have settled for either one at that point. Really, you had to look carefully to catch one of my nods. You had to anticipate it. Here I was, making slight, almost imperceptible movements and hoping the person across from me would pick up on them to save me the trouble of explaining myself or making a series of more considerable, more obvious movements.

When I tried to talk, my voice came out sounding high-pitched and tiny, but more than that, it was a struggle for me to form the words. Here again, my brain wasn't able to get my mouth to voice what it wanted me to say, so my speech was slurred. For a guy who made his living with his voice, this was a big adjustment—and an immediate worry. Inside my head, I felt like I should be able to read the news or interview a celebrity or report the weather, but if I couldn't speak I was nowhere. The effect was like I'd been injected with a little too much Novocain, which made it hard to form words, and then on top of that a little too much helium, which made the words I did manage to form come out sounding like Betty Boop on party balloons. Still, I found very quickly that one very carefully chosen word could communicate most everything I wanted to say, and as long as I could get that word out and have it be understood my eyes could fill in some of the blanks for me. My expression and my soon-practiced subtle gestures could tell the rest, as long as the person on the receiving end of my message was patient. It wouldn't work on television, but it worked just fine for a basic human exchange.

It's hard to accept that your body doesn't work. This is me overstating the obvious, I guess, but it wasn't so obvious to me at first. You can will your body to perform a certain way, and it cannot respond. It certainly took some getting used to. Once, early on, I had an itch I meant to scratch, and I couldn't reach my hand around to get to it. It was the most agonizing, frustrating, devastating, defeated feeling, to be so unable to help myself deal with such a small thing as a simple itch. It made no sense to me. In my head, this was no big deal. In my head, I was healthy. In my head, I was a *fiftysomething* guy who was still something of an athlete, still something of a physical specimen. In my head, my mind and my body were in perfect alignment. But in reality, which was where I was now forced to dwell, the one couldn't control what the other was doing. There was no one in the room but me, and I couldn't call for help. I couldn't even call out in pain or discomfort, because I wasn't really in any pain or discomfort. It was just an itch, after all. I tried to put my mind on something else, but that didn't really help. Then I tried to shimmy in such a way that I could press the part of me that itched up against the sheets, but that didn't really help either. Eventually, a nurse came by and I sheepishly asked if she could help scratch my itch, and she graciously complied, but I hated feeling so desperate, so helpless.

Right away, Dr. Medary encouraged me to think in terms

of what I could do, instead of what I couldn't do. I wasn't ready for rehab just yet—I was still wearing a catheter—but in many ways this was the beginning of my rehabilitation. This would be my new mind-set, going forward, and it was delivered to me almost casually, in an aside, by my neuro-surgeon. It was a tossed-off comment, but I caught it and held it close, as if the rest of my life depended on it—which it most certainly did. So, yes, this was rehabilitation of a kind. This was an important first step.

The all-important second steps would have to wait, be-cause Sand Lake was not really a rehabilitation facility. They weren't set up with all the equipment you typically find in a rehab center—no treadmills, no exercise bicycles, no bal-ance bars. When I was ready, when the blood clot dissipated or stabilized, they would move me to another hospital, where I would begin the long process of recovery. For now, nurses and therapists would come into my room and work my limbs for me, so the muscles wouldn't atrophy, but I was not yet able to do anything physical on my own. I was being fed through a tube, and bathed from a bucket at my bedside. The only thing I could do, really, was psyche myself up for what I was about to face, to consider the new mind-set I would now have to embrace as my own.

I thought of that line from *The Shawshank Redemption*: "You either get busy living or get busy dying." So I got busy living.

My friend Tony and my cousin David got busy first. They pulled out a cribbage board and a deck of cards. I don't know what they were doing with a cribbage board and a deck of cards, but there they were. They thought I could play, so that's what we did. Right there in my hospital room, only a couple hours after I came to. I don't remember that. Tony said I was able to count my cards and keep track of the game, but of course I didn't have the dexterity or the strength to shuffle the cards or move the pegs, so somebody had to help me with that part. I don't remember that either. I also don't remember that everyone in my room was heartened by the fact that I could play cards. Apparently, it was seen as this great indicator of my future recovery, this random game of cribbage. At the time, they didn't know what kind of shape I'd be in. They'd gathered around my hospital bed to say good-bye, not to watch me play cards, but now it looked like I might be sticking around for a while and we could save our good-byes for another day, so this was a good and welcome development.

I wish I could remember who won the game, because I'm a competitive guy, and if I'm going to go to the particular trouble to play a game of cribbage where I can't even hold my own cards or move my own pegs I should at least kick my opponent's butt.

I don't think anyone stayed too long, once I came out of the coma that final time and it became clear to all that I would survive this ordeal. It was not yet clear just how I'd come through it, and in what kind of shape, but they weren't getting rid of me, that much was clear. My family and friends took turns showering me with hugs and smiles and sighs of relief, and then they disappeared back into their own lives.

Nobody wanted to be in the way. My sister Karen stayed on a while longer. Remember, she and Denise had been best friends since high school, so Karen was a big help around the house. She drove Denise the hour or so back and forth to the hospital each day. She was a big help emotionally, too. They cried together, and laughed together, and looked forward together to my full recovery—a recovery that at just that moment was still far from certain. Denise's mom also came down to help out with the kids. She'd been taking care of Denise's Aunt Jean up in Maryland, but as soon as AJ heard what happened to me she told Denise's mom to head down to Florida. She said, "There's nothing you can do for me here. It's not too late for them."

For the most part, though, everyone flew back to their own lives, now that they knew I was going to survive. My brother Chris, for one, had already been back and forth to Maryland before I fully regained consciousness. He had flown down to Orlando immediately on Wednesday, upon hearing the news, and then when he got to the hospital and learned I would be okay he went back home to do his radio show the next day. Then when I took an apparent turn for the worse and Dr. Medary told Denise I might not make it, he came back on Thursday, so I really put Chrissy through his paces. Henry Maldonado, my general manager at WKMG, and Skip Valet, my news director, were at the hospital early and often. I can't say enough about how well they treated me and my family. I had only been at the station for about a year, and they responded like lifelong friends. A great many stroke survivors I've met report that once their bosses learned about their stroke their jobs disappeared. Not mine.

Some of my Sand Lake visitors surprised me. Tom Sorrells, for example, was the WKMG evening weatherman. We were colleagues. We got along great. He'd been a good friend since my first day at the station. And then I looked up one day and saw Tom in my hospital room. This was a surprise—a welcome surprise, but a surprise just the same. You have to realize, the dynamic in the newsroom was that I was the network guy. The others on the WKMG news team tended to treat me a little differently. I didn't ask to be treated in this way, but I had been to the mountaintop, so to speak. I'd been a network guy for so many years. The local guys put a lot of emphasis on that, I guess because I had been where they wanted to go. They put me on a kind of pedestal. I didn't ask to be on any kind of pedestal, and I didn't deserve to be on any kind of pedestal, but that was the vibe I got when I started at the station. And here was Tom, in my hospital room, and my voice was all strange, and my speech was slurred, and I couldn't move, and if he looked carefully he could probably catch a glimpse of my butt peeking out from the flaps of my hospital gown—but still I was thrilled for the visit. It meant the world to me.

My brother-in-law Chris (not to be confused with my brother Chris) also made his presence known. He couldn't make it down to Orlando that first week, but he was like our interpreter for all things medical. He helped us navigate our way through the maze of hospital forms and procedures. He's married to my sister Karen, and he runs a practice of radiologists in Maryland, so he knew his stuff. He talked on the phone with Dr. Medary with real authority, like one of those "I'm-not-a-doctor-but-I-play-one-on-television" characters. This was another good and welcome thing, because he became a real advocate. He asked all the right questions and quizzed Dr. Medary on every decision, and in the end managed to save me and Denise a whole mess of grief. Chris was the one who helped us understand the risks in Dr. Medary's decision to increase my blood pressure. Dr. Medary was able to explain this to us in clinical terms, but Chris walked us through it in real, human terms. He told us what could happen if the blood clot didn't respond the way Dr. Medary hoped it would respond. He was also very patient with us, and helpful in explaining exactly what was going on and exactly what I could expect—from the doctors and nurses on staff, from my health insurance company, from the agencies and institutions that would soon swoop in and take over my care.

I wasn't ready to see my kids just yet. In just a few days, I'd want desperately to see them, but not just yet. I didn't want them to see their dad like this, all weak and nearly paralyzed and knocking on death's door. I didn't even want to talk to them on the phone, because I didn't want them to be afraid of how I sounded. I worried that even if we got past the visit without incident, it might mess with their heads. The twins, Miles and Griffin, were only two years old. They wouldn't understand what had happened, and could only be frightened by my appearance. Denise's daughter, Jenna, who lived with us, was only nine, and it was hard enough to have a stepdad without having to look in on one who couldn't move or talk. I didn't want her to worry about me, or about her mom, which was the more likely prospect. But my own daughter, Maya, was another story. She was ten years old, and lived in New York with her mother, my ex-wife, Judy. Very quickly, I decided Maya was mature enough to handle the uncertainty of the situation. Plus, I really, really, really wanted to talk to her. I was a little selfish, I guess. I wanted desperately to hear Maya's voice, which meant she'd have to hear mine, so I asked Denise to prepare Maya and her mother for how our conversation might go. This was maybe a day or two after I woke from my coma that final time, and Maya had known a little bit that something had happened to her dad a couple days earlier.

When I heard Maya's sweet voice on the other end of the phone I thought I'd gone to heaven. She said, "Daddy!" That was enough to get me to melt—and to thaw some of those frozen muscles. So what did I do? Well, I couldn't leave my little girl hanging like that, long distance, so I started to sing. Anyway, I tried to. Before my stroke, I actually had a halfway decent singing voice. I used to sing to my kids all the time. So I reached into my repertoire and pulled up "Good Night," that great Beatles song from *The White Album*. I hadn't planned on singing, but the song just came. It's the only lullaby I knew. I sang it for Maya when she was small and I sang it now. Anyway, I sang it as best I could. It was probably the most pitiful version of "Good Night" in all of human history, but I crawled my way through it. You could recognize the song, at least. For me, that was saying something. Mercifully, Maya helped me out, and when her voice joined with mine it was a beautiful duet. Of course, it's possible my hearing was all messed up, along with my voice and the right side of my body, but I don't think so. I think we sounded great—so great that I just cried and cried.

Denise didn't let on, but she wasn't at all convinced I would get any better, and a scene like this one must have broken her heart in a dozen new ways, to go along with the couple dozen other breaks she'd already suffered since Tuesday. She was usually a glass half-full kind of person, the opposite of our new lifeline Dr. Medary, but here she couldn't imagine the long climb ahead. Here she could only close her eyes and imagine that she'd be taking care of me for the rest of our lives, and when she was alone she steeled herself against what was to come. But she never let on. When she was with me, Denise gave off nothing but positive, hopeful energy. Everything was going to be okay, she kept saying. This was just a bump in the road. There were no negative outcomes, only positive.

Some months later, Denise told me later that the first time she *really* knew I would come out of this ordeal somewhat resembling the person I was going in was when we were watching *Jeopardy!* one night, just a couple days into my stay at Sand Lake. We were big into *Jeopardy!* in our house. It was like mind-candy, a great distraction. As I wrote earlier, I usually ended my early evenings with *Jeopardy!* before turning in for my 3:00 A.M. morning news wake-up call, but my history with the show ran even deeper. I'd been a contestant on *Celebrity Jeopardy!* on two occasions. I won both times. The first time I played against Robin Quivers, from *The Howard Stern Radio Show*, and Rob Schneider, from *Saturday Night Live*.

On *Celebrity Jeopardy!* you don't play for prize money—not for yourself, anyway. You play for a favorite charity, so I played for Community Services for Autistic Adults and Children, in honor of my younger brother Sean, who's autistic. It's a great organization, and it was a privilege to play for them and call their good works to public attention. My father spent many years on the board, and even served a term as president of the organization, so CSAAC was near and dear to my family. In fact, one of the main reasons I agreed to appear on the show in the first place was the chance it provided to give the organization some publicity and hopefully to win them some money.

The second time I played, I was up against Cheech Marin, from *Cheech and Chong*, and Jerry Orbach, from *Law & Order*. These guys were both tough players, and both were smart and well-read. One of the categories was "Broadway," which isn't exactly fair when you're playing against Jerry Orbach, one of the great song and dance men of his generation. He pretty much ran the category. I remember answering a question correctly about the musical *Rent*, but then Jerry bet big on a Double Jeopardy question about the musical *1776* that would have had me and Cheech stumped. It was a real seesaw battle.

The Final Jeopardy category was "Words." The answer was "*Merrythought*, in old English, is a name for this part of the chicken." I thought, What is a merrythought? Then I thought, Well, it's probably something that makes you feel good. Then I made an educated guess and wrote, "What is the wishbone?" Jerry Orbach made the same educated guess, but I had bet bigger, so I ended up winning another nice check for CSAAC.

On this night, in my hospital room, the Final Jeopardy category was "World War II." The answer was, "FDR, Winston Churchill, and Joseph Stalin met here at the end of World War II." Denise looked at me blankly, but I knew the answer immediately. It was an effort for me to talk, but I had that whole Final Jeopardy jingle to form my answer and put it out there.

Finally I said, "Yalta."

All the contestants got it wrong. Denise turned and smiled at me when the answer was revealed. I smiled back and said, "I still got it." It came out sounding slurred and a little too squeaky and high-pitched for my big body, but Denise understood. And she knew inside that moment that someday she would have her husband back. Up until that time, she wasn't liking our chances. She was looking ahead and imaging what her life would be like without an able-bodied version of me at her side. But now her thinking turned. Now her thinking was, It might take a while, and I might be a little worse for wear, but I was lurking there in that hospital bed, beneath all the not moving and not talking and not being able to care for myself.

I was still me, and so we held on to this one merrythought as tight as we could and hoped for the best. Anything less would simply not do.

I stayed at Sand Lake for a week, and I don't think I left my bed even once. It was too soon for me to begin rehab, but Denise and the doctors began looking into a rehabilitation facility for me right away. I couldn't stay in this hospital room forever. Sponge baths sound nice in theory, but they can be pretty humiliating in a hospital setting, when you're entirely dependent on others for your care. And talk about humiliating? Having to use a bedpan was unpleasant and depressing. Each time, I got to thinking how awful it would be to have to use one forever, so I was in a real hurry to move on from this first phase in my recovery. Plus, in just a few days I'd need to start moving around, to start working my muscles before they failed me permanently. I couldn't count on these nurses and therapists to move them for me indefinitely.

During that first week, I received a constant stream of visitors, probably a few too many as far as the nurses were concerned. There were phone calls, too, only these were difficult for me. I welcomed the connection, but it was an effort for me to talk on the phone. My sister Karen reported later that she tried to ask me questions that required just a one-word answer, because she didn't want me to work so hard to talk to her. I thought that was considerate of her, but what I didn't know was she would hang up the phone and cry because she could only ask her big brother "yes" and "no" questions.

This was a good example of our own McEwen form of rehab, because it wasn't only me who needed rehabilitation. So did everyone around me. Denise, my kids, my dad, my siblings...everyone had to adjust how they were around me, to absorb these changes to my abilities and help me take them in stride. Even my friends and colleagues had to adapt. People don't talk about rehab for loved ones and caregivers, but they probably should, because if I had caught any negative or sorrowful vibes from my friends and family it would have set me back. And if the people I loved didn't make the extra effort to help me avoid certain obstacles or pretend these obstacles didn't exist, I would have undoubtedly grown even more frustrated at my situation than I already was. That's probably one of the reasons why I didn't encourage Denise to bring Miles and Griffin down to see me right away, because it would have been devastating for me to see myself in my little boys' eyes. Forget how *they* would have responded to me. I was worried how *I* would respond to them seeing me helpless and bedridden.

But I wouldn't be helpless and bedridden for long, I determined. Already, I was the one guy in ten who managed to survive my particular kind of stroke. Next I would be the one guy in ten who manages to make a full recovery. After that, I would return to work and to the rest of my life. Anyway, that was my plan, and there was no talking me down from that plan. I was completely focused on it. That's why a lot of the details of those first few days at Sand Lake are a little murky, because I was so dialed in to what was in front of me I couldn't really pay attention to the details. I couldn't tell you what I ate, or what I talked about with my doctors and therapists. I couldn't tell you exactly what I did during that long stretch of days. All I could tell you was what was right in front of me.

LIFE BEFORE STROKE: *RADIO DAYS*

moved from that Beverly Hills youth hostel to an apartment in North Hollywood, and from there to a small house in Reseda, but it's not like I was moving up. I was just moving. Looking back, I think I was a little too sensitive to be a comedian. If the audience didn't laugh at one of my jokes, I took it personally. This is not a good thing, if you want to do stand-up. You need a thick skin. Sometimes the same joke kills one night and dies the next, so you can't take it personally. You have to figure out what works, and what doesn't, and move on from there.

Back then, in the late 1970s, Jay Leno was working the Playboy circuit and making about $300 a week. That was big money to us up-and-coming comics, and there

I was reaching for it, and reaching for it, and I was earning just enough to keep ahead of my rent. Each month, it was a scramble. Me and my stand-up buddies, we'd sit around and talk about what it would be like when we finally made it. I started out extremely confident, and now I didn't think I'd ever make $300 a week doing stand-up. I could make that much moving furniture, or working in a bank, but that's not what I wanted to do. That's not why I left school—or, why I went to California in the first place.

When I finally pulled the plug on my stand-up career, it was with a heavy heart. I wasn't a quitter, but I was a realist. I took the same view years later, when I was in rehab, when people were telling me I might not regain my abilities after a certain stretch of time. Still, I refused to give up on myself, because no one could prove to me that I wouldn't achieve my goals. In my stand-up career, though, it started to seem like I was beating my head against the wall. The longer I worked at it, the more my goals seemed just out of reach. I never minded taking the stage for a 1:00 A.M. slot at some comedy club, but I wasn't going to be the next Cosby or Pryor, that much was clear. It was time to do something else. I drove an old Volkswagen in those days, and I packed it with my worldly possessions and headed east. I think I cried all the way from California to Denver. And then, somewhere in the Midwest, those tears turned to resolve.

Somehow, I landed that first job at that Baltimore station, and soon I landed a bigger job at a bigger station in a bigger market. That's the career path I'd chosen, so as much as I liked being back in Maryland I had no choice but to follow it up and out. I moved to WWWW-FM in Detroit. I thought to myself, Detroit? When you're starting out, you don't stay in any one place for too terribly long, and you can't afford to be too picky when a good job comes along. You bounce around, from station to station, until eventually you stick. I went to Detroit thinking it would be part of the bounce, not part of the stick.

Everyone in Detroit referred to the station as the W4, because of the call letters. There was a deejay at the station named Sky Daniels, who worked from 6:00 P.M. until 10:00 P.M., and I followed him from 10:00 P.M. to 2:00 A.M. Together, we went from third to first in the ratings in just a few months, but it wasn't without effort. I was at the station twenty hours a day, sometimes. I didn't mind. I was young. I was single. I could have stayed in Detroit indefinitely, I suppose, if the station wasn't sold out from under me. That's another thing you have to deal with in radio. There's almost always a change in management or some other change in direction before long. It's not the most stable industry. Every job feels like the job you have for the time being, the job you take to get you to the next job.

Another thing I learned early on about radio is that

it's a small business. *Very* small. If you work with someone in one market, chances are you'll work with him or her again in some other market, in some other capacity. It's a boomerang industry, because everything comes back to you sooner or later. That's what happened here. Twice. The sales manager at W4 would go on to become the general manager of a station in New York, and he helped me get my big break there. But that wouldn't happen just yet. First I had to get my big break in Chicago, at WLUP-FM, "The Loop," which was probably the hottest station in the country at the time. There was a lot of buzz attached to The Loop just then, only I didn't really want to go to Chicago. I was an East Coast kinda guy. The East Coast meant home, but my old partner Sky Daniels had been working at WLUP, and then he became the music director there as well, and when a spot opened up on the 10:00 P.M. to 2:00 A.M. shift he recommended me. I thought, I guess I can give Chicago a try.

The Loop was a blast. It was a real rock 'n' roll station. Chicago was a blast, too. There were great restaurants, and interesting neighborhoods. I felt at home in Chicago, and the deejays at WLUP were like rock stars. They made public appearances and emceed at concerts. We used to do these live remotes, and hundreds of listeners would turn out, sometimes thousands. We played these big, anthem-type rockers like "Highway to Hell," by AC/DC, or "Won't Get Fooled Again," by The Who, and when the chorus came around I'd turn down the

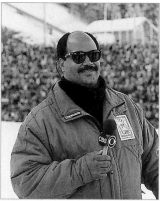

Mark broadcasting from the Winter
Olympics in Albertville, France, 1992.

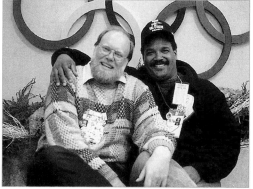

Mark posing at the
Winter Olympics
with Kevin Coffey.

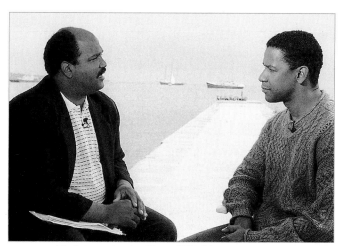

Mark interviewing Denzel Washington on a pier
in Cannes, France, 1992.

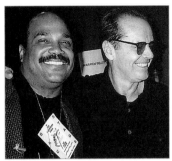

Mark with Jack Nicholson, backstage at President Clinton's first gala at the Capital Centre, 1993.

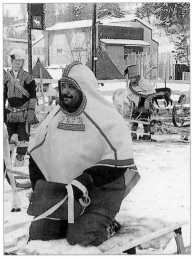

Mark preparing a segment for CBS on a reindeer sleigh in Lillehammer, Norway, 1994.

Colin Powell, Mark, Paula Zahn, and Harry Smith on the set of *CBS This Morning*, 1995.

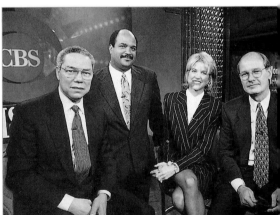

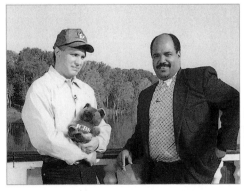

Mark interviewing Garth Brooks onboard *The General Jackson* in Nashville, 1996.

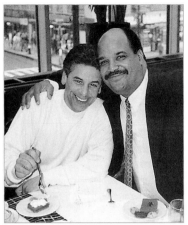

Tony Mirante and Mark in
New York City, 1996.

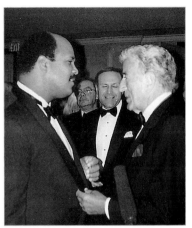

Mark interviewing Tony Bennett
in Washington, D.C., 1997.

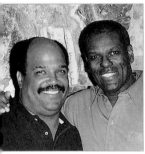

Mark and Hall of Fame pitcher
Bob Gibson, 1997.

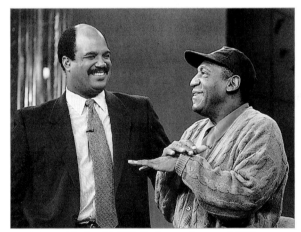

Mark with Bill Cosby on the set of *CBS
This Morning*, 1997.

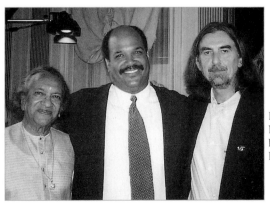

Ravi Shankar,
Mark, and former
Beatle George
Harrison, 1997.

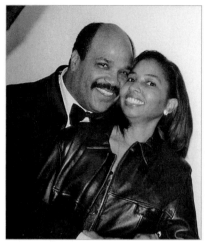

Mark with Cathy Black, Entertainment Producer at CBS's *The Early Show,* for the Grammy Awards.

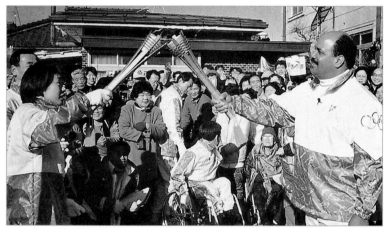

Mark running with the Olympic Torch at the Winter Olympics in Nagano, Japan, 1998.

Whoopi Goldberg and Mark on the set of *CBS This Morning,* 1998.

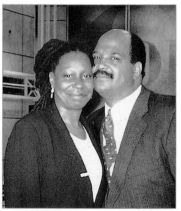

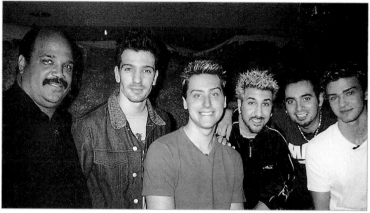

Mark and the members of *NSYNC, 2000.

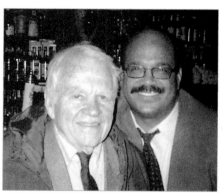

Andy Rooney and Mark at his going away party from CBS's *The Early Show* in New York, 2003.

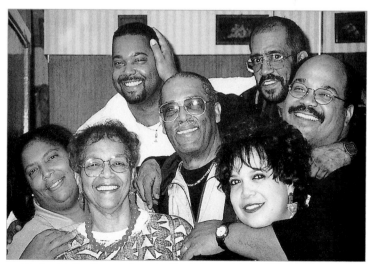

Mark with family members Leslie, Dolores, Chris, Alfred, Karen, and Billy, before his stroke.

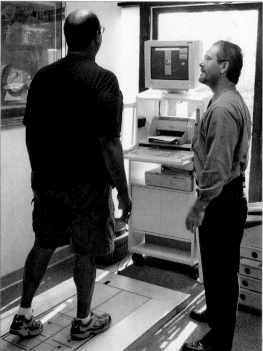

Mark working out with Rod Olson, the head of BIRC and his first physical therapist there, 2006.

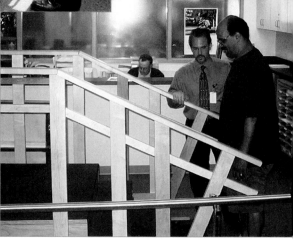

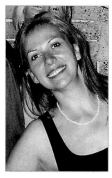

Tommi Ann Wilde, Mark's speech therapist.

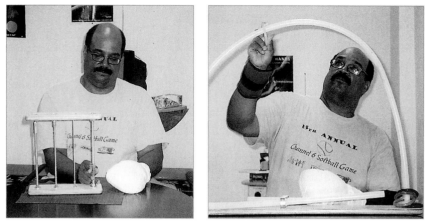

Mark doing constraint therapy in Lady Lake, Florida, 2007.

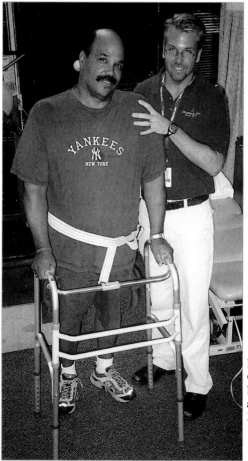

Mark with Walter Caldwell, who taught Mark to walk again, at the BIRC center, 2007.

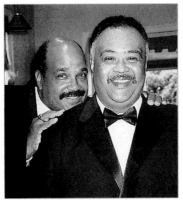

Mark and his best friend,
Tony Colter, 2007.

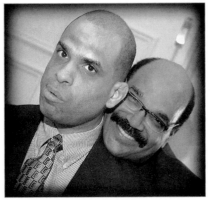

Mark and his brother Sean.

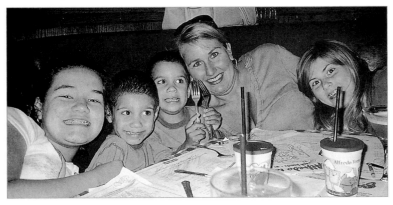

Mark's wife, Denise, and their children: Maya, Griffin, Miles, and
Jenna in Florida, 2007.

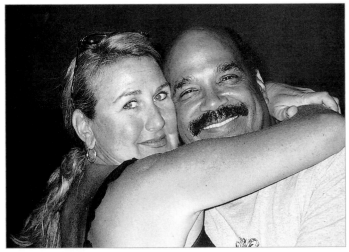

Denise and Mark, 2007.

vocal on the soundboard and hold the mike out to the audience so they could sing along. To the listeners at home or in their cars, it sounded like they were missing out on a giant party—and they were. No other deejays were doing that kind of thing at the time, and soon everyone was doing it.

My first contract was for $35,000. They offered only $30,000 to start, but they asked me to act as the station's research director along with my on-air responsibilities, and my dad told me to go back and ask for an extra $5,000 for the research job. The general manager of the station was a guy named Les Elias. He just smiled when I put it to him the way my dad suggested, and said, "I think we can do that." This was 1980, and $35,000 was a lot of money. I lived in a nice part of Chicago, with a nice car. I looked up one day and realized I loved what I was doing. The paycheck. The lifestyle. The part how they treated us deejays like rock stars. I even loved my 10:00 P.M. to 2:00 A.M. shift. It's a different feeling, being on a rock 'n' roll station in the late evening hours. Your listeners are home, or kicking back with friends. They're not racing to get from one appointment to the next, or tuning in for some distraction at work. They're listening because they want to hear some good music, or they want in on some great party.

I was playing an album one night, late, and took a call from a listener. She sounded nice. Her name was

Linda Boston. Linda Boston, from Chicago. I loved her name, and I teased her about it. We talked for a long time. A lot of times, listeners would call in and we'd get to talking, so this wasn't unusual. Late at night, we welcomed the distraction. It helped to pass the time during some of the long album cuts we used to play.

After an hour, Linda said, "Maybe we should meet."

Denise and I weren't together at this point, and it wasn't clear to me that we would be together anytime soon, so this seemed like a good idea. We were broadcasting from the Hancock Center, on the 37th floor. It was around midnight. I was still on the air when Linda arrived. I sent an intern downstairs to let her in. I wasn't looking for a girlfriend, but there she was. We got along great. Linda was pretty and intelligent. We dated for the whole rest of the time I was in Chicago, so I always tell people who like to call up radio stations to be careful. Deejays, too, I tell them to be careful about the calls they take. You never know where that kind of call might lead.

I was only at the station a couple months when I hit number one for my time slot. Sky Daniels was on in front of me, doing the 6:00 P.M. to 10:00 P.M. shift, and he was number one in his time slot too, and we thought we were pretty cool, taking our shows to number one in two cities, back to back.

But this was radio, so our run didn't last too long. A new program director came in, and the way it goes is the new guy wants to bring in his own lineup. He looks to shake things up, and in the shaking I was pushed to overnight. In radio, overnight is the graveyard shift. It's where program directors put their on-air talent with the big contracts if they don't want them on during the rest of the day. There's no question, this guy wanted me to quit. At any other time in my life, I might have done just that, but I was liking this new relationship with Linda, and I was liking Chicago, and there was no place else I wanted to be. My friends at the station were always asking me if I was quitting, but I sucked it up and worked that overnight shift. I wouldn't let station management push me out until I was ready to leave. Somewhere in there, our overnight numbers improved, and soon the station moved me to mornings. They couldn't get rid of me, I guess.

I liked working mornings. That's usually where a station puts its marquee show, where it pulls its biggest numbers, and I did pretty well in the mornings. Program directors liked me in that time slot because I'm a bright-sounding person. Not bright, as in intelligent. Bright, as in cheerful, sunny, wide awake. Like a morning person.

All of a sudden, things went from bad to great. They'd tried to push me out the door, and I kind of hung in the doorjamb for a while until they invited me back in, and now I was the face of The Loop. The face, the voice, the whole upper body. Now I was the morning guy. Now I had a news reader, and a traffic and weather person, and the chance to develop some regular segments and characters and bits and whatever else it is that morning radio guys do. I got a raise. For the first time in my stop-and-start career, I'd allowed myself to think I made it. Or, at least, that I was on my way.

LUCERNE

Following You, I'll Climb a Mountain

My memory kicked in about a week after my stroke, when I was transferred to Lucerne, an Orlando rehabilitation hospital. Everything before that is all bunched together. I remember bits and pieces, but I was in and out of consciousness so often during those first couple days that it took some time for me to get any kind of clarity or continuity. Even now, all these months later, there are whole chunks of time that are still lost to me. It wasn't until I got to Lucerne, really, that the fog from my stroke began to lift. Before that, I don't think I could have told you what day it was, or what was going on in the rest of the world.

It was a weird, uncertain time. It was almost otherworldly,

to be completely out of it one moment and back in it the next. It wasn't just my semiconscious state that left me uncertain. It was also a tough adjustment, coming to grips with the fact of my stroke and the uphill climb ahead. It's a lot to handle, especially when your thinking is still clouded and your head feels like it belongs to someone else. It's a funny thing, the way the mind works, the way it can fit events and circumstances that don't normally go together in a way that makes sense. Not funny in a "ha-ha" sort of way, but funny in a disorienting way. At least, this was my experience, as I started to heal and figure out what was going on with me, but it was also my experience that I had moments of absolute confusion. During these moments, nothing seemed to make sense. The lucid moments I did have that first week at Sand Lake were mostly filled with trying to navigate my way through a mess of information on brain injury and such. I still didn't know too much about stroke, and I still thought someone must have made some kind of mistake in my diagnosis. I kept coming back to this one point in my thinking, as if a different word attached to my condition would somehow change my situation.

Lying there in my hospital bed, waiting for my full-blown rehabilitation to get under way, I learned a couple things. I started to pay attention. There was nothing else to do, so I guess I figured I'd do well to tune in to whatever it was that was going on. I learned a couple things more, on my long road to recovery, but I took in new information on a need-to-know basis at first. I focused on what would help me going forward. I learned that one hundred and sixty thousand Americans die each year as a result of stroke, but underneath that alarming figure was a more important number as far as I was concerned: another five hundred thousand *survive* a stroke. This was key, not least because this group now included yours truly. Believe me, I was thrilled to be among this survivor group, but it also scared me because it turns out that surviving a stroke is the number-one risk factor for having a second stroke. According to Dr. Patricia Davis of the University of Iowa Hospitals and Clinics, the increased risk of having a second stroke within five years after the first is about 30 percent. I tend to take a positive view on such things, but here I took these statistics to mean I might have been spared, but only for the time being.

I was both lucky and cursed, I guess. Once again, I was stuck on that word. *Lucky.* Yes, I was lucky to be one of the five hundred thousand survivors, but now it appeared I was consigned to a lifetime of significant risk and worry that another stroke would find me before too terribly long. Out of nowhere, I had to start paying attention to my "risk factors." These can come in two types among patients prone to stroke. There are modifiable risk factors, which are things you can change or control, and which include conditions like high blood pressure, heart disease, high cholesterol, and type 2 diabetes, along with lifestyle causes such as smoking, obesity, and drinking to excess. Fortunately, I didn't have to worry about too many of these, except as I've mentioned I did suffer from high blood pressure, like almost everyone else I knew in television news. I also struggled with my weight, from time to time, but I carried it on a big frame, and I was in reasonably good shape.

·Then there are nonmodifiable risk factors, such as age, gender, type 1 diabetes, and a family history of stroke. These, of course, I couldn't do anything about, but here again I counted myself lucky, because as far as I knew I was in the clear on these fronts as well. There was no family history of stroke, and no personal history of diabetes. I couldn't do anything about my age or gender, although here too I was in the relative clear. At fifty-one, I was still on the young side in terms of risk. In a couple years, I'd be at greater risk, because according to the American Heart Association Web site, the chance of having a stroke more than doubles for each decade of life after the age of fifty-five.

For reasons doctors and researchers cannot conclusively determine, stroke is more common in men than in women. However, more than half of all deaths due to stroke occur in women, which suggests that the effects of stroke are more devastating in women than in men.

The only big risk factor working against me was race. According to the National Stroke Association Web site, African Americans are twice as likely to die from a stroke as Caucasians. The rate of first stroke in African Americans is almost double that in Caucasians. Indeed, African Americans are more susceptible to stroke than any other group. There are some explanations for this. For one thing, one in three African Americans suffers from high blood pressure, so since that risk factor is more prominent it follows that as a group we're more at risk on this front than any other racial group. Also, African Americans tend to have a higher incidence of obesity and heavy smoking, so these factors play into it as well. And sickle-cell diseases, which tend to strike African Americans with far greater frequency, can cause blockages in the blood vessels that can often result in a stroke.

Drug and alcohol abuse have also been linked to a higher incidence of stroke, and there's even some evidence to support the theory that strokes are more common among low-income groups than among high-income groups.

I determined to focus on the modifiable risk factors within my control. From here on in, I vowed, I would watch what I ate and exercise regularly, although at this early stage I was still a long way from even irregular exercise. Still, it was yet another reason to will myself back to whole, as quickly as possible, to keep myself healthy enough to ward off any future stroke.

I also learned about TIA—or, transient ischemic attack. I'd heard the term kicked around during my stay at Sand Lake, but never took the time to understand it until I was a little more settled. Realize, it was never made clear to me that I had suffered a TIA on my way to the major stroke that nearly did me in, but it surfaced in my research as one of the more common types of strokes, and one of the most under-reported. According to the American Stroke Association, a TIA can produce stroke-like symptoms that usually resolve with no lasting brain damage. TIAs are also known as "warning-strokes" or "ministrokes," although it's important to note that the majority of strokes are not preceded by a TIA. Of the people who have suffered one or more TIAs, more than a third will suffer a subsequent stroke. Common symptoms of TIA include numbness or weakness in the face, arms, or legs, especially on one side of the body; sudden confusion and difficulty speaking or understanding; sudden trouble seeing in one or both eyes; sudden trouble walking; sudden dizziness and loss of balance and coordination; and sudden and severe headaches. These attacks are relatively short in duration, and they leave no permanent damage, which is the main difference between TIA and stroke.

The causes of TIA are a reduced blood flow at a narrowing artery to the brain; a blood clot in the heart or some other part of the body, which can travel to the brain and block an important blood vessel; and a narrowing in one of the small blood vessels in the brain that can momentarily block blood flow. The blockages can be caused by a condition called thrombosis, which is basically the formation of a clot within a blood vessel; or by an embolism, which is the term to describe the movement of a clot from another part of the body to the brain. It can also be caused by a condition known as stenosis, which describes the severe narrowing of an artery leading to the brain, or an artery in the brain itself.

The National Institute of Neurological Disorders and Stroke reports that since there is no way to tell whether stroke-like symptoms are occurring as a result of an acute stroke or a TIA, patients should assume the former and seek emergency treatment. They should not simply assume that the symptoms will go away.

Over the next few months, as I began my rehabilitation and became more and more involved with the people at the National Stroke Association and the American Stroke Association, I learned that even though there are approximately two hundred and forty thousand cases of TIA reported in the United States each year, the actual number is estimated to be several times that—meaning, that most of these events go undetected. I also learned that every stroke is a life-and-death emergency, and that not every stroke patient reports experiencing every symptom. Some symptoms go away and then return. Some symptoms never show up. The bottom line here is that if you are experiencing any symptoms, you should seek help immediately.

As I write this, there's an exciting study out of London that confirms the importance of quick and aggressive treatment of a TIA or ministroke. Oxford University researchers found that patients treated within twenty-four hours of a ministroke can reduce by 80 percent their chances of having a more serious stroke in the next three months. The lead author of the study, Dr. Peter Rothwell, helped to put this number in perspective. He said, "We normally get excited about ten to fifteen percent." He also said that minor strokes should now be classified as medical emergencies.

Back to me and my rehab. Emotionally, I was a little all over the place. Don't get me wrong: I was thrilled to be alive, given the events that had played out in my brain, and blessed to be surrounded by such caring and supportive friends and family. I understood that, even though everything else was a muddle. I also understood that I was determined to work my way back to how I was. But underneath all of that I was also scared and stubborn and tentative and confused and probably a little angry, too. It was a strange mix of emotions, and what was particularly unsettling was that I was unable to articulate what I was feeling. I can't stress this enough. There was no place to deposit all those runaway emotions, because my body wasn't working well enough to put them into words and download them onto someone else, so there was a kind of bubbling frustration going on inside my head. It felt like I was about to burst.

Typically, Denise and I would talk about everything. Whatever we were facing, whatever we were worried about, we'd deal with it together, but here I couldn't even manage to tell her what was on my mind. It was a maddening thing, to be so plugged in (at certain moments) to what was happening and yet at the same time to be so hopelessly unable to express myself. It's like I was watching my life play out behind a two-way mirror from a soundproof room, like I was there and not there all at the same time. I was a participant and an observer, all at once. I could see and hear and understand everything that was going on around me, but it was hard to get anyone else to see or hear or understand me. This was a huge handicap, let me tell you, and I wasn't at all prepared for it. Another stroke victim described the sensation as what it must be like to be buried alive, but that only gets close to the frustrating weirdness of it. It explains how many stroke patients feel trapped by their bodies, but it doesn't get at the rest of it. Better, it's like watching a movie of your life, without having a part in it.

I went to Lucerne because it was affiliated with Sand Lake. I wasn't really involved in this decision—that was mostly Denise's call, with some input from Dr. Medary—but as I came to understand it, there wasn't much of a decision to be made. It was the obvious place for my rehabilitation. It was in downtown Orlando, which was a good thing as far as Denise and the rest of our family were concerned, because Sand Lake was a haul from our house. It used to take Denise almost an hour, sometimes longer if there was traffic. The commute was starting to get to her. Lucerne was a lot closer, so it cut way down on her time away from the kids when she came to see me.

I checked into Lucerne under Denise's maiden name because I was well-known from my time on CBS. Someone at the hospital suggested this, because they didn't want to have to lie if someone called the hospital switchboard asking for me, and it turned out to be a good idea. I was Mark Bosies instead of Mark McEwen, but I still got a lot of strange looks and comments. People would say things like, "You look a lot like that guy Mark McEwen from television." I'd usually smile and say, "That's me." It didn't really bother me. It was just an extra something I had to learn to accommodate. In the beginning, of course, I didn't say much of anything because it was so difficult to talk. Here again, that's one of the things I had to learn to deal with, not being able to say exactly what I wanted to say, exactly when I wanted to say it, even if it was something trivial like a joke or an aside. It changes the way you look out on the world. And it changes your personality. You get an idea in your head, or you're participating in a conversation, and you have to stop and weigh the extra effort in communicating that thought or idea. Most of the time, I didn't even bother, because it was just too much trouble. Or I'd edit what I had to say down to the smallest phrase possible to make myself understood, and I'd leave it at that, and even then I couldn't always get my point across.

I saw a young man in the dayroom one morning who'd lost his leg in a horrible car crash. He was in a full body cast, and there were tattoos everywhere the plaster didn't cover. He was a big Dallas Cowboys fan. I didn't want his injuries, or his diagnosis, but I liked how nobody bothered him.

I met an old guy down the hall who'd just had hip replacement surgery, and a woman across the way who was also recovering from stroke and who was still unable to walk. They were also left to do their own thing, in their own time, in their own way. I liked that, too.

The folks at Lucerne did a great job respecting my privacy. Even the other patients were good and kind in this regard. I had no reason to complain about anything. Nobody really bothered me the whole time I was there or treated me any differently than anybody else. As for us patients, we treated each other with warmth and mutual respect, and we cheered each other on as we began to chart our progress. But in those first couple days, when my health and well-being were a looming unknown and out of my control, I was reaching for whatever measure of control I could reclaim, and just then privacy and anonymity sounded pretty good.

This was a small point, after all. The big point was the stroke itself, and what it had done to my body, and what I would do about it. I was a wreck, basically. What I would do about it was everything in my power, but at just that moment I was essentially powerless. For nearly a week at Sand Lake, I had been on a bedpan and catheter. I had to be bathed and fed and dressed. I could barely move the right side of my body—and as I've written, moving the left side was no cakewalk, either. It hurt to talk, and to swallow. Some days, it even hurt to breathe. And every movement I did manage was deliberate and methodical and frustrating. Exhausting, too. Some movements, I had to completely relearn, like I was an infant learning to walk for the first time. Others, I had to learn to do in a completely new way, like feeding myself with my left hand instead of my right, or dialing a telephone.

Still, I looked around at all the other Lucerne patients and decided they were worse off than me. In truth, I was probably worse off than most of the patients on my unit, but I was in denial. This happens a lot with brand-new stroke patients, I soon learned. This was my brain working a little too hard to compensate for the rest of me that wasn't working too well at all. A part of me thought that this was happening to someone else. Another part of me convinced myself I was merely tired, and that my strength would return to my right side after I got some rest. It didn't seem real to me, because my new reality was so far removed from my accustomed reality that I couldn't reconcile one with the other. There was probably another part of me, deep down, that thought I could just close my eyes and wish all my troubles away.

You have to realize, I had always been the guy who could do whatever he wanted to do. I could be funny. I could be smart. I could be athletic. I could be fast or slow. But now I could only move at one speed—*really* slow. Now I could just forget about being funny or smart, because the best I could hope for was to just make myself understood. The way I was—the *old* Mark—was just out of reach. Every gesture, every movement, every response was suddenly very, very difficult, and some of the most basic and familiar movements and abilities seemed impossible. It must have been heartbreaking for Denise, to see me struggling and to imagine a lifetime at my struggling side, but she never let on.

One of the great finesse moves Denise made during this

time was to keep my kids from seeing me for as long as possible. It's mostly in retrospect that I think of it as a great move, because at the time, of course, I was desperate to see them as soon as I transferred to Lucerne, but Denise knew I wasn't ready. She knew it would be devastating for me—and for them. In the beginning, at Sand Lake, I was in no shape to see them, and I knew enough not to press for it, and to bend to others who suggested I wasn't ready to do so, but I started asking to see them once I moved to Lucerne, once I started moving around a little bit. Every time I asked, Denise kept coming up with perfectly reasonable explanations for why the kids couldn't come that particular day, without ever telling me what she was really up to. With my daughter, Maya, who was all the way up in New York, it made sense that it took a week or so for her to make arrangements to fly down to Florida, but with our twins, Miles and Griffin, and with Denise's daughter, Jenna, it was a little tricky. They were right there in Orlando, and I was anxious to see them, but Denise very subtly put off their visits until she thought we were all ready. This one had a doctor's appointment on the other side of town. That one had a playdate after school. There was always some piece of plausible juggling, and Denise reported it in such a way that I never really noticed she was dragging her feet, and I look back now and think, Good for her.

That first visit with my kids was a meaningful moment. Actually, it was a meaningful moment and a nonevent, all at the same time. The kids were like, Hey, Dad, where have you been? Kids are funny that way. Here we'd been apprehensive about how they'd react, and it just rolled right off of them, seeing me in that hospital bed. Miles had a little trouble with it, but not too much. With twins, it often goes that one of them is more closely connected to their dad and one is more closely connected to their mom. Miles was mine. He'd never seen me at anything less than full strength. With the boys, I was the kind of dad who got down on the floor and wrestled and goofed around, but here I was just laying there, not doing much of anything. Miles seemed kind of mad about that. He actually ignored me, for the first few minutes. But Griffin couldn't climb up on my belly fast enough, and he started reaching for the television remote and the button that adjusted the bed and all the other interesting new stuff that was around the room, and soon his brother was joining him. They were barely two years old, and they were bouncing up and down on the bed, on me, like it was some big adventure. And Jenna was just so happy to be there. She was fascinated by the wheelchair in the corner of the room, and she sat in it and wheeled herself around, and it didn't seem to bother her in the least that I was in such bad shape. I mean, I'm sure it bothered her. She would have rather seen me fit and healthy. But she wasn't traumatized by the situation, the way we'd feared. She was perfectly content to roll around in the wheelchair, visiting with her family, and for a moment I could close my eyes and listen to the joyful sounds of our children and imagine that everything was back to normal.

Maya didn't come for another week or so, and that visit went a little differently. That was more emotional. Maya's always been very protective of her parents. She's an old soul. She worries about me when she's with her mother; she worries about her mother when she's with me. And here she seemed to go into caregiver mode. She was only ten years old, but she was attentive and compassionate. It probably terrified her to hear me speak, and it must have really freaked her out to see how hard I had to struggle just to move or perform the simplest tasks, but she never let on. Denise had prepared her for this, but it's one thing to know your dad is in bad shape and quite another to see him in bad shape. And yet to Maya's great credit, she just smiled and held my hand. I think back on this now and I'm so overwhelmingly proud of her, for keeping it together the way she did, because inside that moment, with Maya just standing there and holding my hand, was all the motivation I needed to get better.

At Lucerne, my neurological care was now in the hands of Dr. Nicholas Bagnoli. Dr. Medary signed off on my case when I left Sand Lake, although I continued to see him from time to time, and I remain forever grateful for his role in setting me right. Dr. Bagnoli checked in when I checked in at Lucerne, after my condition had stabilized, so I never really had the same relationship with him. They wouldn't move me to a rehab facility until I was stable, so it was never about life and death with Dr. Bagnoli, the way it had been with Dr. Medary. The blood clot in my brain was no longer a worry, so there wasn't a whole lot for him to do. Nothing against Dr. Bagnoli, but the crisis had passed, and now all that was left was to repair the damage. Of course, this last was no small thing, but we were no longer in crisis mode. We had moved into crisis recovery. This cast a woman named Tommi Ann Wilde as the real point person for my care at Lucerne, and for the balance of my rehabilitation. Tommi Ann was my speech therapist, but she was a lot more than that. Very quickly, she became like a lifeline, in almost every aspect of my care. She became my friend, my coach, my biggest cheerleader, and my most demanding taskmaster. She was the point person for every aspect of my rehabilitation. My speech was the one area where she worked with me in a hands-on way, but Tommi Ann consulted with me on my physical and occupational therapy regimens as well. She was in my ear and in my head the entire time I was at Lucerne, and she's been there for me ever since.

One of the first things I knew and liked about Tommi Ann was that she was a big Bon Jovi fan. I thought, Anyone who likes Bon Jovi is okay by me. She had seen them perform live nine times. I had my own Bon Jovi memory to share. At WAPP, the first New York rock station I worked at, Bon Jovi won our homegrown talent contest. They won with the song, "Runaway," which became one of their first big hits. Tommi Ann certainly knew the song. She knew everything there was to know about Bon Jovi. She had a friend she talked on the phone with all the time, and when I caught snippets of their conversation it always seemed to be about Bon Jovi. She was hard-core—but then, there was a time when I was pretty hard-core about rock 'n' roll, too. We talked about music all the time. At first, Tommi Ann did most of the talking and I did most of the listening, but I think she used the common ground of rock 'n' roll as part of my speech therapy. She was pretty clever, when it came to pushing me. She found ways to get me to do the hard work she put out in front of me without me realizing it was hard work.

In her spare time, Tommi Ann worked as a bartender at a club inside the arena where the Orlando Magic play. I thought it was the perfect job for her, because she was such an energetic, outgoing person. She really seemed driven to help her patients, like nothing was more important. By the time we met, she was already thinking of leaving Lucerne for a position at another rehab facility, but she stayed on an extra couple months to work with me—and I'm eternally grateful that she did.

I've spoken to a lot of stroke patients in the past year and a half, as well as to survivors of other types of trauma, and almost all of them tell me there was a voice in their heads encouraging their recovery. For some, it was a parent or a partner or an influential coach or mentor. For others, it was an inspirational line from a movie or a song. For me, Tommi Ann was that voice. If something appeared difficult or insurmountable, I'd close my eyes and imagine Tommi Ann talking me through it. She was such a great motivator that I could feel the power of her persuasion even when she wasn't around. I'd be about ready to give up on something, and I'd think, What would Tommi Ann say if she knew I was thinking about quitting?

My days at Lucerne were built around Tommi Ann's visits. Let's be clear—my speech therapy sessions weren't necessarily a highlight, because they came to represent hard work and frustration, but they were a focal point. Tommi Ann came to see me every afternoon at 4:00. That was our standing time. Sometimes it seemed like everything that happened before 4:00 was just me spinning my wheels until Tommi Ann got there and we got to work. Sometimes it seemed like everything that happened after she left was just me winding down and getting some rest so I'd be ready for her visit the next day.

At first, I was so weak that speech therapy was all I could really handle, and even that was tough. I also did physical therapy, but I didn't make a whole lot of progress in this area right away. (Occupational therapy would kick in a couple weeks later, when I left Lucerne and started working at another facility on an outpatient basis.) I was used to seeing results whenever I worked hard at something, so this was an adjustment. There would still be results, but they would come on their own schedule. Or, sometimes they'd come and I wouldn't even notice. With the speech therapy, though, I was able to push myself and start to see some results almost as soon as Tommi Ann and I began working together. She started me out identifying the different shapes my mouth needed to make in order to produce different sounds.

It sounds like a simple thing, but trust me, it's complicated. And grueling. We laughed a lot—in part, because it made the hard work pass a bit more easily, but also because we developed the easy rapport of true friends. There was a lot to laugh about: my predicament, Tommi Ann's predicament, trying to get me to do things my body had no interest in doing, and on and on. She even had me moving my tongue in a circular motion around my lips, to strengthen my tongue muscles, and every time I did that particular exercise I hoped like hell no one was watching me. After working with Tommi Ann, I was constantly thinking where my tongue needed to be, relative to the roof of my mouth. She had me thinking of the various shapes associated with various sounds, things I never had to think about before. She had me doing all these different exercises, and they were draining. We didn't even bother with words during our first few sessions, just sounds. The hard *k* sounds, I remember, were especially difficult. The *s* sounds, too. Over and over, we'd work on these sounds, until eventually we graduated to words.

For homework, I'd have to hold up a mirror and watch my tongue form the desired shape as I read through a list of words. *Clock, spaghetti, scarecrow, sister, sand, steer, sea, carrot, keep, keel, compact*...I had to say the words just right, or Tommi Ann wouldn't let me move on to the next thing. She'd come in and say, "Do you want the spaghetti now?" This was her way of getting me to respond. I couldn't just nod, or grunt an assent. I had to answer her back in a full sentence, making sure to emphasize my speech on the word *spaghetti*. I'd have to say, "Yes, I want the spaghetti now." Of course, there was never any spaghetti, and there were times when I would have paid dearly for a plate of fresh, home-made pasta, instead of just another mouthful of frustration, because Tommi Ann's *spaghetti* was just a collection of sounds. She had all these little sentences worked out for me, to force me to speak the most difficult words, with the most difficult sounds. And then there was the casual con-versation between us, and this also played a key role in my therapy. She'd tell me a story about one of her favorite Bon Jovi concerts, and then I'd feel compelled to join in with a story of my own, and in the extra effort it took for me to tell it were the fruits of all those long, hard hours in speech therapy.

I really wanted to tell Tommi Ann about the first inter-view I got to do when I started working at CBS. I didn't have the strength or the voice to tell Tommi Ann the full story, but I tried to get it out anyway: I'd been hired as the weath-erman for the morning news program, but underneath that job description was the promise that I'd get a chance to in-terview pop culture celebrities from time to time. For a while, it seemed that loose promise might never amount to much, but the producers all knew about my background as a rock 'n' roll deejay, so when Tommy James came to town for a show they looked to me to do the interview. It was a giant thrill. I'd interviewed tons of musicians over the years, but never on television—and this was *network* television, to boot. Of course, by the late 1980s, Tommy James was essentially an oldies act, but he'd still produced some classic cuts from rock's golden age, like "Mony, Mony" and "Crimson and Clover."

I was looking forward to meeting him.

In network television, I was learning, nothing was left to chance. There were segment producers whose main job was to make sure the three- or four-minute interviews they arranged went off without a hitch. They did all the legwork. They even wrote down a couple pages of suggested questions, which someone handed to me just before the show. Frankly, I was more nervous about reading these prefab questions and following the segment producer's script than I was about conducting the actual interview, and I guess my floor manager (and now great friend) Tony Mirante was able to pick up on this. He came over to me during a break and said, "Don't worry about those questions, Mark."

I was so green, so new, so young, so eager to please my new bosses that I was prepared to read down that list of questions if that was what my segment producer wanted, but Tony said he wouldn't do that if he were me. I held up the questions and said, "So what am I supposed to do with these?"

Tony said, "Forget about them. They're just suggestions. Ask him what you want to know."

It was the single best piece of advice I ever got at CBS. *Ask what you want to know.* And I was reminded of it when I was working with Tommi Ann. Because she loved rock 'n' roll almost as much as I did. Because she was smart enough to know when to toss out the script and improvise. Because she saw each of her patients as individuals, with particular strengths and needs and interests, and because she was somehow able to harness those strengths and needs and interests. Because she didn't waste her time or her patients' time, following a set routine or list of procedures.

Of course, I couldn't tell Tommi Ann my Tommy James story the way I wanted to just yet, but she listened patiently while I tried. Before I started working with Tommi Ann, I'd never realized how much of your fine motor skills come into play just to say a few simple words. Man, it was hard. And tiring. But Tommi Ann was relentless. She didn't understand the meaning of the word *quit*—which, as best I can recall, was never on our list of words. It had that hard *k* sound Tommi Ann liked to stress, but it was such a negative word that she probably avoided it for that reason alone. She was always very positive. Tough, but positive. She's one of the most upbeat people I've ever met, but underneath that good cheer was a drill sergeant.

Tommi Ann set the bar high and expected her patients to rise to meet it. If I told her I was tired, or if I couldn't do a particular exercise or make a particular shape with my mouth, she'd pretend not to listen. She'd say, "Just one more time, Mark." Or, "Just a few minutes more." Or, she'd just go ahead in such a way that I had no choice but to follow. I could be tired later, she'd say. In her mind, on her watch, everything was just within reach, whereas before I met her everything seemed so far out of my grasp. It was a seismic shift in perspective that was undoubtedly essential in my recovery, and I credit Tommi Ann for that.

After just a couple sessions, I found myself looking forward to Tommi Ann's visits each day at Lucerne, probably because it was easy to see the results of all that hard work. Like I said, it wasn't a highlight of my day, but it was very clearly the focus. The other thing I looked forward to was Denise's daily visit. This was a true highlight. Denise usually came right after my session with Tommi Ann for dinner. During the first week or so, I think I squeezed in a nap between my session with Tommi Ann and my visit with Denise. I napped a lot, during that time. I was always tired. After a while, though, I cut it down to just one nap during the day, but I was still pretty tired. It takes a lot out of you, all this therapy. Already, the stroke had done a number on me, and before I could regain my strength they had me working double-time trying to get my body right.

The food at Lucerne was nothing special, but Denise always made it a point to bring me something from home. Her visit alone was already a high point, but the care package put it over the top. She had some help in this area. Our friends and neighbors took turns with our care and feeding, for a stretch of several weeks just after my stroke. It was an incredible kindness. Really, I can't say enough about these good people, and each night at six or seven o'clock, I couldn't say anything because I was too busy enjoying whatever it was they'd cooked up for us that evening. The women in our neighborhood, they set up a rotation and took turns cooking for Denise and the kids. It was one less thing for Denise to worry about, putting a hot meal on the table, and there was always enough for a goodie bag for me. Whenever I heard Denise's footsteps outside the door to my room, my first thought was, Alright, Denise is here. My second thought was, Alright, I get to eat real food!

For that week or so at Sand Lake, I didn't have much of an appetite, but that may have had something to do with how weak I was at the time. It was difficult to chew, and for the first couple days it was painful to swallow. There were a lot of liquids, as I recall, and soft foods like Jell-O and pudding. After that, they tried to get me to eat solid foods, but it wasn't so easy. Once my appetite returned, it was hard to get excited about hospital food, which was why it was a great, good thing the way our neighborhood pals kept those homemade meals coming our way.

There was a lot of downtime at Lucerne, so I asked Denise to bring me a Walkman and some of my CDs to keep me company. I'd always been a big reader, but reading was also hard at first. I had *The New York Times* and the *Orlando Sentinel* delivered at home, and Denise brought them to the hospital when she came to visit, but I didn't really read them those first few days. They just piled up on the shelf by my bed. I couldn't hold the newspaper still enough to read, because my hands were so shaky. Even such a simple task as turning the pages was difficult. Later on, I was able to thumb awkwardly through the newspaper—at least well enough to glance at the front page and take in some of the headlines, and to read the sports pages to see how my Yankees were doing.

I also tried to read books, with only a little success at first, but I was determined to get back to it straightaway—probably before I was fully ready. I asked Denise to bring in some James Patterson novels, because he tended to carve his books into short chapters. It seemed more manageable to me. I don't think I understood too much in the beginning. The part of my brain that recognized and processed language still wasn't firing on all cylinders, and it was difficult to follow a complicated plot. Also, I had a hard time with homonyms like *object, produce, close,* and *read,* words that are spelled the same but can be pronounced and interpreted differently. For example, you can hold an *object* in your hand, and you can *object* to a situation. You can be *close* to something, as in near, and you can *close* (or shut) a door. You can *read* in the present tense, and you can just finish having *read.*

These subtle distinctions were very confusing to me, and they came up a lot. You'd be amazed how often you encounter words with double meanings or multiple pronunciations over the course of a typical day. I know I was. This is especially so when you're not conditioned to take them in. There's a part of your brain that's become conditioned to processing these types of distinctions without any effort at all, so most of us catch these double meanings without even thinking about them. But not me. I had a hard time with them. Also, I had a hard time concentrating well enough or long enough to read for any longer than a few minutes, so for the time being that left music. I wasn't an iPod or an MP3 player kind of guy. (That would come later, thanks to a gentle push from my daughter, Maya.) It took me just about forever to give up my precious LPs for CDs, so for the time being it was still just an old-fashioned CD Walkman for me. Denise brought in some Al Green, some Little Feat, some Springsteen. I put on my big, old-fashioned headphones and tried to drown out the other sounds on the unit. There was always a lot going on at Lucerne, and it was sometimes hard to relax after a particularly difficult session, but the music helped. Once again, I could close my eyes and imagine I was the old Mark, spinning rock records for some radio station.

Somehow, I could still hear Tommi Ann's voice beneath my headphones. Her message would get through. This was the power of her personality. Even when she wasn't there, she was there. She took the word *wrong* out of my vocabulary. Whenever I struggled, I'd reach a point where I'd throw up my hands and say, "I'm doing it wrong." And then she would say, "No, you're not. You either do it correctly, or incorrectly, but never wrong."

One of Tommi Ann's big things was to compare the progress her patients were making to the progress you'd make on a diet. She said that if you do the work you'll see results, but you might have to look hard for them. Then she reminded me that when you're trying to lose weight you don't see the results from day to day. You might not even see them from week to week. But others can see them. If you don't see someone for a couple weeks, and they're motivated about dieting or therapy or whatever it is, you can really see a difference each time you meet, but when you're the one doing the dieting or the therapy it's not so easy to chart your progress. The changes can be subtle, gradual. Plus, with a diet the pounds can fall away pretty quickly at first, and then you reach a plateau and the trick is maintaining that weight loss and from there finding the will to lose even more. It works the same way with therapy, Tommi Ann said. Speech therapy, physical therapy . . . it's all the same. You can make a bunch of progress, and then slow down and start to think you're not getting any better, but you need to find the will to stick with it and make even more progress.

You need to persevere.

LIFE BEFORE STROKE: *THE APPLE*

f I was from Chicago, I probably would have stayed at The Loop and become a local fixture, but a part of me was itching to get back to the East Coast, so when I read about an opening at a station in New York I was all over it. There was a front-page notice in *Radio & Records*, announcing that WAPP-FM in New York was looking for a morning team. I wasn't part of a morning team, but I was a morning guy. I figured if they liked me, they could pair me with some other morning guy and then they'd have a team. I also figured I could get an interview, because the sales manager from W-4 in Detroit, Pat McNally, was now the general manager there. He took me to lunch at the 21 Club, one of the city's most famous restaurants. I'd never been to 21.

We got drunk, drunk, drunk. We talked about radio, and the people we knew in common. We talked about WAPP, which they were calling The Apple. It was a new station, part of Doubleday Broadcasting.

After lunch, I walked back to my hotel. I went the long way around, because I wanted to clear my head. It took me about a half hour to walk just a few blocks. By the time I got back to my room, there was a message from Pat, with his home and work numbers. There was also a message from the program director, Dave Hamilton, with his home and work numbers. I thought, Hey, I think I got this job.

Within a week or so, WAPP hired a guy named E. J. Crummey to be my partner. He was from Boston. I was from Baltimore, by way of Detroit and Chicago. I guess the thinking was we could meet in the middle and make a good team. Dave Hamilton offered to match what I was making at The Loop. I was so anxious to go to New York that I agreed to his opening terms. I didn't have an agent at the time. I just had my dad down in Maryland.

E. J. called me up and said, "Mark, you're a terrible negotiator." I was costing him money, because they'd offered him the same salary, but I just wanted to get to New York. I apologized to E. J. and said, "We'll renegotiate as soon as we hit number one."

I went to Linda to talk about the job. She knew I wanted to get back to New York. She knew that if we were meant to be together we'd find a way to make it work, so she encouraged me to take the job. Then I went to the program director at The Loop to tell him I was leaving to take the job in New York. He said, "Sure you are." He couldn't believe it. I was on the number one station in the country, on the number one morning show, making good money. This was the same program director who tried to get me to quit the year before, and now he wanted me to stay.

E. J. Crummey and I were on the cover of *Radio & Records*, to announce the launch of our new show, which was to be called *The Crummey-McEwen Show*. The name was my idea. I thought it made it sound like a bad McEwen show. We started in the fall of 1982. They put us on a couple overnights, just so we could get familiar with the board. My mom and dad came up to New York for our trial run. They stayed in a midtown hotel. They stayed up that first night, to hear my debut. The first song I played was "Rock This Town," by the Stray Cats, which I thought was appropriate.

The station itself was pretty run-down, somewhere in Queens, but the signal was strong. It covered the whole metropolitan area. My parents were pretty impressed. They didn't know a whole lot about radio. All they knew was that their son was about to be introduced as the cohost of a new morning radio show in New York.

Eventually, Linda came to New York, too. We decided

to get married. We got married in Maryland, in my parents' house, so I began this new partnership in my private life at the same time I was beginning this new partnership in my career.

Life was looking pretty good.

Crummey-McEwen turned out to be a successful team. We did a lot of call-in bits. These were becoming a kind of staple in morning radio, but we liked to put our own spin on things. One morning, we interviewed Nelson Doubleday's mechanic. We thought it would be funny, to talk to someone else who worked for the same boss.

E. J. said, "What's Nelson like?"

The mechanic said, "He's a pisser."

E. J. hit the seven-second delay button, but I thought we should let it slide. Our bosses told us to sound like we were from New York, and "pisser" sounded like we were from New York, so I said, "Let him say what he was going to say." Then we asked the mechanic again what Nelson was like and he repeated that he was a pisser at parties.

At one point, the mechanic said, "I do all of Nelson Doubleday's cars, and I also do his daughter's car."

E. J. responded, "Do you also do his daughter?" It was a cheap line. It was also regrettable.

As soon as the show ended, E. J. and I were called in to the office of Gary Stevens, the president of Doubleday Broadcasting. It felt like we were back in high school, being called in to the see the principal. I thought that what would probably happen was E. J. would be reprimanded, or fined, or suspended, or otherwise disciplined for his remark, and that I would be reprimanded, or fined, or suspended, or otherwise disciplined for being his accomplice. But this guy Gary Stevens was furious. I thought he'd have a heart attack, the way he was yelling at the two of us. He ended up firing me, although E. J. was allowed to stay on. It made no sense, but that's how it played out.

I'd only been at The Apple for about three months. I was a couple weeks shy of a severance clause in my contract. Pat McNally, to his great and lasting credit, found a way to wait until one day after that date to get around to firing me. He kept me on a kind of suspension, until he finally had to let me go. It was a nifty bit of maneuvering and loyalty that saved me a $14,000 severance payment. It took some of the sting out of my firing.

As it turned out, it would be another loyal turn from another WAPP colleague that would take me to my next gig—at WNEW-FM. There had been a deejay at WAPP named Ken Dashow, and he left for WNEW about a week before I was fired. We'd only worked together a short time, but we'd become friendly. Ken heard what happened and called me immediately. He said they were looking for people at his new station. He set up a meeting for me with Scott Muni, who was a legend in New

York radio and a pioneer of the progressive rock radio format. He also had one of the most distinctive voices in radio. It sounded like he was gargling with gravel, but it sounded just right on him. He knew everybody in music.

I'd only been in New York a short time, but everyone I knew listened to Scott Muni. He was like a god to us deejays, so I was a little alarmed when he called. He said he was doing double duty as program director and was looking for experienced deejays with a sense of humor and a sense of rock 'n' roll history. I thought he was kidding. Or, I thought maybe it was one of my friends, doing his voice and putting me on. A lot of people in New York radio could do a passable impression of Scott Muni, including Billy Joel, who did it for me years later in an interview, so this last made a lot of sense. But it was really and truly Scott Muni, and for some reason he really and truly wanted to get together. We met at a bar called The Quill and Quiver, just across from the *Daily News* building. He called me "Fats." I thought, Maybe I need to go on a diet. Then I learned he called everyone "Fats."

We went on an epic bar crawl. Back then, Scott used to drink Scotch. I drank Heinekens. We went from bar to bar, from neighborhood to neighborhood, depleting the city's supply. We started in the early evening, and we kept on well into the night. When one place closed, we went out in search of another. I don't know how we managed to pick ourselves up and keep moving, but we managed. Scott would knock on the door of a bar after it had closed, and the bartender would know who he was and open the door for us.

At the end of the long night I thought, Hey, I think I got this job. I couldn't remember where I'd parked my car, but that didn't matter to me just then. I'd been on a legendary bar crawl with the legendary Scott Muni, and things were looking up.

REHAB

Try, Just a Little Bit Harder

A typical day at Lucerne began at six o'clock in the morning. That's when the nurses woke me up to take my blood pressure and give me my medication. I couldn't stand being woken up so early. This must sound surprising, coming from a guy who made his living in the early morning hours for the longest time, but I was so tired from all that therapy and from the beating my body had taken as a result of my stroke that I couldn't keep my eyes open. It got to where I could almost sleep through this early morning visit, because it was still the middle of the night as far as I was concerned. I'd stick my arm out; they'd take my blood pressure, give me my pills, and leave. Then they'd turn out the lights, and I'd go back to sleep. It's like my alarm was set for six, and then I reached out and hit the snooze button for another couple hours.

At ten minutes before eight, my sister Karen would call on her way to work. She was like clockwork. This was usually my first phone call of the day. Sometimes, it was my wake-up call. They woke me up for good at about seven-thirty, but sometimes I drifted back to sleep. Most times, though, there was so much noise and activity on the unit that I'd be wide awake when Karen called. She'd say that she was on her way to work and so was I. That's how I'd come to look on my rehabilitation, like it was my new job. Looking back, I think that's really how you have to approach rehab, like it's your full-time gig. I used to wear a suit and tie to work, and now I wore gym shorts and sneakers. Also, now I had an easier commute, because my work came to me when my therapists would meet me at my room.

These were the phone calls I wrote about earlier, where Karen very thoughtfully tried to steer the conversation in such a way that I only needed to offer one word in response.

Are you feeling good today?

Yes.

Are you going to have breakfast?

Yes.

Have the kids been to visit?

No.

I never realized at the time how much extra effort Karen put in at her end of these conversations, just so I wouldn't have to put in too much on my end. My whole family was good about that. My father called every day, too, only he called at all different times. The phone in my room could only receive incoming calls, so I came to look forward to these calls from friends and family. It was my one-way connection to the rest of the world, to a life that had been momentarily set aside by stroke. The extra effort my father put in was to call every day and to make sure he found a way to mention how good I was sounding each day, how much better. He didn't have to say anything, but he made sure he did anyway. My dad and I are pretty close. We share ideas, thoughts, concerns. Right after my stroke, my voice was high-pitched, and tiny, and each day my father would say it sounded like it was coming down. He said I sounded stronger, better. I told him early on to be honest with me, and not to sugarcoat things. He told me early on that one thing he hated was people who kept the truth from him, under the guise of being nice. So he was honest with me. He was my father, but he was as good a friend to me as I've ever had. I valued his opinion about my voice, because he was a voice coach. He taught opera. He sang in the choir at church. He knew what he was talking about.

When I was at CBS, my dad joined me for an appearance on a late-night show I was hosting called *The Midnight Hour*. That was a real thrill—for both of us. He sang a song called "Here Comes That Rainy Day" with Patrice Rushen, the Earth, Wind & Fire horn section, and Jeff "Skunk" Baxter on guitar. They sounded great.

Before the show, the executive producer came to tell me the song was too long. He said, "It's four minutes! We wouldn't give Sinatra four minutes."

I said, "*You* go tell my dad."

The executive producer sought out my father backstage and said, "Mr. McEwen, the song is too long. There won't be any time left for you to talk to Mark on the air."

My father said, "With all due respect, I can see my son anytime. I came here to sing."

And he did.

At Lucerne, I found myself looking forward to my dad's daily calls. He sprinkled them at all times throughout the day, so it was always welcome to find him on the other end of the line. It put a dash of surprise into my otherwise predictable routine.

At eight o'clock, another nurse would come in with a tub of hot, soapy water, a washcloth, and a small towel for my bath. Maya called it a cowboy bath. Back in Maryland, it's a sponge bath. The first time Maya came to visit, she saw the tub and the washcloth and said, "Hey, a cowboy bath!" Then she left the room, to give me some privacy. It didn't matter what you called it. Sponge bath, cowboy bath...it was just a daily reminder that I could no longer do for myself, and the perfect motivation at the start of each day to get up and get moving again. When you're healthy, a nice sponge bath can be a real treat. When you're disabled, it can be a symbol of your disability.

Breakfast was sometimes difficult, especially in the

beginning, because I was relearning how to feed myself. I had to do it with my left hand. I had no strength at all in my right hand. I couldn't even hold a fist, so you could just forget about utensils. My left hand was already weak because it wasn't my dominant side, but my right side was also weakened by the stroke, so I couldn't really cut anything with a knife, or butter a piece of toast, or bring a cup to my lips without spilling. I had to lean in and sip from a straw, and eat only soft foods. It was an effort, and an ordeal, and there was no real payoff at the other end because it was just hospital food. If it had been a nice juicy steak, maybe it would have been worth all the trouble.

After breakfast, I started in on my physical therapy. For most of the time I was at Lucerne, I worked with a terrific guy named Walter Caldwell. There were other physical therapists, but Walter was a constant. He was a good-natured tyrant. He's about 5'11", with sandy blond hair. He runs marathons. He used to be heavier, before he took up running. He never mentioned that he used to be heavier, but I heard this from the other therapists. Remember, I had some difficulty talking, those first weeks and months after my stroke, but I could hear just fine. I mention his marathon running here because it's a good indicator of Walter's relentless work ethic. He's the kind of guy who just puts his head down and moves ahead, and when you work with him for a while you start to adopt the same mind-set.

We worked a two-hour session each morning, and Walter really put me through my paces. Walter's sessions were grueling, like Tommi Ann's, but in a different way. I was still in a wheelchair when I got to Lucerne, but Walter's mission was to get me up and moving as soon as possible. Even if it was just for a couple steps each day, he wanted me out of that wheelchair. I was extremely unsteady on my feet, but he encouraged me to go for it anyway. He used to have me walk down the hallway, wrapped like a mummy with these moving-man ties they used to help us keep our balance. The ties were like those harness-leashes you sometimes see parents use when they're teaching their kids how to walk, to keep them from darting out into traffic or disappearing in a crowd. Walter had me wrapped up good and tight, and he'd walk right behind me, making sure I didn't fall as I teetered down the hall. It was a tremendous effort just to go fifty feet, and there were a couple times when I lost my footing and nearly went down, but Walter kept pushing me. With his encouragement, I went from a wheelchair to a walker to moving about on my own steam in just a couple weeks.

I'll never forget the first day I managed to walk the length of the hall outside my room, all by myself. No wheelchair. No walker. No harness-ties. Just me. I was so overcome with emotion and accomplishment that I cried, and when I told Denise about it later, she cried too. Underneath those tears there was the bittersweet notion that my life had been reduced to a series of small, negligible tasks, accomplished with great effort, and I wonder now if that was maybe part of the reason I was so quick to cry. The tears were tears of triumph and joy, but somewhere in the mix there were also tears of frustration. I dreaded the thought of a lifetime reduced to a series of small, negligible accomplishments—and yet at the same time I dreaded the thought of a lifetime without them.

Between physical therapy in the morning and voice therapy in the afternoon, my days at Lucerne were fairly full—and unbelievably tiring. You can't imagine how exhausting it can be, relearning the common, everyday motions and actions we don't even think about performing. Walking. Talking. Reaching. Grabbing. Lifting. It was like a boot camp, just to get me back to where I was. I can still picture myself at the wrist-exercycle they had in the physical therapy room at Lucerne. I'd never seen one of these contraptions before. Essentially, it's an exercise bicycle you operate with your upper body. I had to do revolutions for fifteen minutes at first, to strengthen the shoulder muscles on my right side, the side which was most affected by the stroke. If the flywheel mechanism on the thing didn't have its own momentum, I don't think I could have completed five minutes, but somehow Walter saw me through to the full fifteen, and soon after that I worked my way up to a half hour.

Walter and the other physical therapists also had me doing leg-lifts on the mat—a routine I was familiar with from my high school wrestling days, only back then it was no effort at all. Here at Lucerne, I could barely complete my initial sets of fifteen without a total feeling of agony and helplessness, and yet here, too, I got over the initial fatigue and worked my way up to sets of thirty—another small triumph on my growing list of small triumphs.

I was so unabashedly proud of myself, for the good, hard work I was doing at Lucerne. I looked around and saw that I was better off than most of the other patients. There weren't too many of us—only ten or so. I think it was designed as a small unit, so the therapists could get the most out of their patients. There was a lot of attention, a lot of encouragement. The therapists created a super-friendly, informal atmosphere, in which we were meant to go about the hard, monotonous work of putting our bodies back together. They pumped in music for us as we worked out, and for most of the time I was there the radio station played Christmas music. I don't know about you, but I've always been a big sucker for Christmas music, especially rock 'n' roll Christmas music. It really got me going. I used to play a lot of the songs when they first came out, like the Eagles' "Please Come Home for Christmas," and what I didn't help introduce on the radio I grew up with, like Ronnie Spector's "wall-of-sound" covers of Christmas classics, so I felt a special connection to the music.

Some of these songs, you hear just a couple notes and your toe starts tapping, so the music was a great motivator. Plus, it made me smile.

We patients stuck together and cheered each other on. There was the spirit of the Christmas season, which accounted for some of the good cheer on the rehab unit, but it was mostly about the *esprit de corps* of all of us being in the same fight, trying to retake the same hill. Most of the other patients were recovering from hip or knee replacement surgery. Most of the patients were older than me, but there were some who were considerably younger. There were other stroke patients, too. There were a lot of wheelchairs sprinkled around the workout room. There was one guy who always wore a Big Dog T-shirt his kids had given to him, and another guy who had lost one of his legs in an accident. We never really learned each other's names or backstories, but there were familiar, friendly faces all around, and we greeted each other warmly each morning. Sometimes, it was just a quick nod or smile, but there was meaning to it. There was an unshakable sense that we were all in this thing together, whatever *this thing* turned out to be.

I always marveled at how hard these other patients worked, at how nobody ever really complained. I took my cue from them. I didn't complain either. Not to Walter. Not to Tommi Ann. Not to any of the other therapists I worked with on the unit. Sometimes I'd complain to Denise at the end of a long, hard day. Sometimes I'd despair that I was never going to fully regain my ability to walk, or to tie my own shoes, or reclaim my seat in the anchor chair at WKMG. Sometimes I'd just moan about how tired I was. But that was just frustration. The truth was, I loved the hard work. I loved how it provided an outlet for all the pent-up energy

I had no place else to put. And I looked forward to making a full and complete recovery. Anything less would simply not do.

We worked out until an hour or so before lunch, but before we could eat we had to go to Group. This was interesting. In the beginning, we sat around in chairs grouped in a kind of semicircle, and did group stretching exercises with large rubber tension bands. The idea was to stretch after our strenuous morning routines, to give our muscles time to recover, and to provide a time in a group setting for us to unwind and decompress. Sometimes we talked as we stretched, and sometimes we didn't. First we worked our arms, and then we moved to our legs. The therapists would count off for us, and we had to follow their count.

Over time, I came to regard Group as the capstone to my rigorous morning. It was something to look forward to. The hard work of physical therapy was behind us for the day, so this was like a victory lap. We patients were warriors, grouped in a loose semicircle, stretching out the kinks from our difficult morning battles, each of us fighting our own separate battle but somehow linked by this group exercise and our shared experience.

Some of the people at Lucerne knew who I was and what I did for a living. Others did not. I didn't mind it either way, because the folks who did recognize me from television were careful to respect my privacy and to treat me like anyone else on the unit. To the folks who didn't recognize me, I was just another patient on the unit, doing his thing. I didn't call attention to myself, because that's not my nature, but there was one time when I just couldn't help it. Attention called itself to me. I received a get well letter from President Bush. The *original* President Bush—or, "41," as he is sometimes known. One of the aides on the unit recognized the return address and said something to me as I opened the mail, so it became a kind of curiosity. I was curious, too, because I certainly wasn't expecting a letter from the president.

I first met President Bush at the Cheeca Lodge in the Florida Keys. We were scheduled to do an interview the next morning, and were seated next to each other at a dinner the night before. He was seated between me and Chris Evert. He couldn't have been more gracious or charming. Our interview the next morning went extremely well. He was considerate, and insightful, and personable. Afterward, I gave him a CBS News hat, and he joked that he could get into any press conference he wanted to, as long as he was wearing the hat. It was the first of four interviews we did together, and each one was more revealing than the one before. I liked him enormously.

Once, long after President Bush had left office, Texas A&M University hosted a father-son presidential exhibit, on the campus where he would locate his presidential library. President Bush wasn't doing any interviews before the event, which was to commemorate the presidencies of John Adams and John Quincy Adams, and George H. W. Bush and George W. Bush. However, everyone at the *Early*

Show saw it as an event of great historic significance, and the producers asked me to reach out to President Bush directly. They knew we had struck up a friendship and thought perhaps I could land an interview on the back of it. I hated to mix my personal and professional lives in this way, or to put a friend in a difficult spot, but I made the call. And sure enough, the president's office called back an hour later with a time and place for me to do our interview. We were the only news organization to feature a one-on-one interview with the president ahead of the Texas A&M event.

When my sons were born, my friend the president sent the boys a letter on his Kennebunkport stationery. It said, "I used to be president, but now I'm like your father and just a proud dad." I thought it was such a warm, generous gesture, so I wasn't at all surprised when I received this handwritten letter from him while I was at Lucerne. I was thrilled, and curious, but I wasn't surprised, because President Bush had shown himself over the years to be a warm, generous guy, the kind of guy who sends get well cards to his friends. In this one, he apologized for his wiggly handwriting, and wished me a full and speedy recovery. It meant the world to me. I showed it to Dr. Bagnoli, who happened to be making his rounds when I opened the letter, and he just about fainted.

After Group came lunch, and after lunch a well-deserved nap. I don't know if all the other patients napped after lunch, but I certainly did. Each day, I was more exhausted from the workout, more exhausted from the aftereffects of my stroke, more exhausted from the weight of what my life had become—but it was the good kind of exhausted. It was the kind of feeling where sleep comes quickly, and even just an hour's nap leaves you feeling well-rested and refreshed.

My time at Lucerne was marked by a series of firsts—and each one was fairly emotional. I can still remember the first time I went to the bathroom on my own. Man, what a simple pleasure. When they finally took out my catheter, I felt like a free man, and then when I was able to graduate from the bedpan to the bathroom—first with the help of a wheelchair, and soon after that with a walker, on my own steam—it was like I'd been toilet trained. I wanted to shout it out from my hospital window and let the world know I'd gone to the bathroom by myself, but thankfully I held off on this kind of celebration.

Instead, I called Denise.

My first shower was another milestone. There were grab bars and other things in the bathroom to help me out if I felt unsteady on my feet. And believe me, I felt really, really unsteady on my feet. This was especially dangerous on a wet bathroom floor, where I could have easily slipped. But I was determined. The therapists were very, very strict about letting us go into the shower unattended. They didn't want us falling down and setting our rehab back. The first time I had permission to shower on my own, I shuffled into the bathroom and turned on the water. I moved really slowly, with extreme caution, because of course I didn't want to fall. Once again, I caught myself crying. There I was, standing beneath the spray, crying like a big baby because I was finally able to do something for myself that had been way beyond my ability just a couple weeks earlier.

Shaving was another matter. I don't think anyone even bothered to shave me when I was at Sand Lake, or if they did I was too out of it to take note, but Denise brought my razor from home when I got to Lucerne, and she was able to clean me up and keep me looking presentable. The doctors suggested I use an electric razor at first, so I did. It would be some time before I could shave myself with a straight razor, because even I wasn't foolish enough to put a razor in my unsteady hand, but when I finally got around to it I managed just fine, although it felt a little bit like I was taking my life into my own hands.

Probably the most memorable *first* came on my first trip home. Somehow, Denise had arranged for me to leave the hospital on a day pass after I'd been at Lucerne a couple weeks. Already, the talk had turned to the time when I would finally be sent home for good, so everyone thought it would be a smart move for me to try on the outside world for an afternoon. It had been almost a month since that ambulance had picked me up at the curb in front of the airport and taken me to the hospital, so I was looking forward to this like you wouldn't believe. I'd never felt so cooped up in my life, and I looked on that day pass like one of those Get Out of Jail Free! cards you get in Monopoly.

For a couple days leading up to this big event, I was working on clearing the last hurdle I'd need before they let me out, even for this one day. The deal was I had to be able to walk over uneven terrain. I don't know if this was the hospital's rule, or my therapist's rule, but it was something I had to do. By this point, I'd mastered the flat, polished floors of the hospital hallways, and I'd even become fairly expert on the wet tile floors of my bathroom, but walking outside was still tricky. There could be cracks in the pavement, or rocks underfoot. Or if you're walking on a path, there could be undulations and protruding tree trunks and all kinds of other obstacles, so Walter took me outside during our sessions to get me up to speed. He took me outside with my walker and steered me toward what looked like particularly treacherous ground but was really just a garden path. Then he told me to start walking. I didn't do so well with my first couple steps, but I got it eventually. I managed to walk a hundred yards or so without falling down, and when I was finished Walter said, "Good job, man. You're ready."

Denise picked me up in our minivan, and I got in and turned up the radio. "Real Love," by the Doobie Brothers, was playing. Then I rolled down my window and stuck my head outside to take in the air as we drove. I was like a playful puppy, sticking my head out the window. (At first, I was going to say that I was like Peter Fonda, hitting the open road in *Easy Rider*, but it's impossible to look cool like Peter Fonda when you're sticking your head out the window of a Toyota Sienna minivan.)

For some reason, the breeze was an absolute thrill. I couldn't get enough of it. I looked around, and everything seemed brand new. Being in the car seemed brand new. It was just a minivan, but it was the ride of my life. The Orlando skyline seemed brand new. The midday traffic on the freeway. The streets of our neighborhood. Walking through the front door of our house.

Everything was as if it was the first time.

I was deliriously happy, but I was also ridiculously tired, so I went directly to our bedroom to lie down. The boys were out with the babysitter. Jenna was with her dad. Maya was in New York with her mother. We had the house to ourselves. For some reason, our bed struck me as being unusually high. It's true, our bed frame is higher than most, and it was certainly higher than the hospital bed I'd gotten used to these past few weeks, but it was an effort for me. I couldn't sit down on the bed, I had to climb onto it. Denise climbed on the bed next to me. We watched television for a while. We cuddled. Denise always kept a lot of pillows on the bed, and that's one of the things I remember most from that afternoon, all those pillows. There were pillows everywhere. If I wasn't careful, I would have been swallowed up by all those pillows.

Anyway, we cuddled, and it had been a long, long time since we had cuddled together like this, and all during that long, long time I'm sure we each took turns wondering when we'd find ourselves in this kind of intimate situation again. We even talked about it, a little. At times, the idea of making love had been the furthest thing from our minds and at other times it was probably one of the only things we could think about—as much for the simple pleasure of the act itself as for what it represented about our lives going forward.

Well, you can probably guess where I'm heading with this. I'm not the sort of guy to kiss and tell, but I will offer up some of the juicy details here because I think it might be helpful to other couples going through some of these same motions. Denise and I ended up being intimate that afternoon. We didn't plan on it, and I wasn't even sure I was medically cleared for sexual activity, but it just happened. I was moving slowly, but I was moving. I wasn't quite the old Mark, but I was pretty darn close. Denise was afraid she might hurt me—and, quite frankly, so was I. But we managed just fine.

For whatever reason, I cried after making love, the same way I cried after taking my first shower, and walking my first hallway, and every other post-stroke milestone I experienced. I was just a bundle of raw emotions, and a big crybaby. Denise cried, too, only here we were both crying happy tears. After that first big sign that I would be okay, that night we were watching *Jeopardy!* in my hospital room, this was the next indicator that we would someday be back to normal. So it was a good and welcome thing, and our tears reflected that. We weren't quite there yet, but we were getting there.

As it turned out, I had no business resuming my sex life just yet. I could have killed myself, apparently. (It's a helluva way to go, don't you think?) I didn't say anything to my doctor or to any of my therapists or nurses at the time, but a week or so later, when it came time to check out of Lucerne, the subject came up. I was going over some of my aftercare dos and don'ts with one of the nurses, and there on the list of not-just-yets was sexual intercourse. I wasn't sure I was reading the list right, so I said, "Do you mean it's not okay to make love?"

The nurse said, "No. I'm afraid you'll have to wait awhile longer. It's still too soon. It's possible you could have another stroke."

So I said, "I'm afraid my wife and I have already done it."

The nurse looked at me aghast, and said, "Mr. McEwen, you're not supposed to do that here!"

"Oh, no," I said. "Not here. It was at home. In my own bed. When I was out on a day pass."

The nurse smiled. I think she was embarrassed at how she reacted when she thought Denise and I had been having sex in my hospital bed. Now that we were just two consenting adults in the privacy of our own home, it wasn't so bad. But there was still the matter of another stroke. I certainly didn't want that day-pass session to be our one and only intimate moment going forward. I said, "How long do I have to wait before it's safe to make love to my wife again?"

The nurse said, "Do you live in a house with a staircase?"

I nodded.

She said, "When you can walk up those stairs without

any trouble and without any shortness of breath, then you should be okay."

That's all I needed to hear. All of a sudden, I was Jack Nicholson in *Something's Gotta Give*. Remember that scene, where Keanu Reeves tells Jack he can have sex again after his heart attack when he can walk up the stairs from the beach to his house?

Old Jack pretty much raced up those stairs straightaway— and so did I.

LIFE BEFORE STROKE: WNEW-FM

I n the early 1980s, WNEW-FM was probably the coolest rock station on the planet, the epicenter of FM radio. We played classic rock, only back then we didn't call it classic rock. It was just rock.

I started at WNEW in 1983 as a fill-in deejay. Eventually, they put me on overnights, where I learned that New York is like no other market in radio. In New York, the overnight shift is still the graveyard shift, but at least there are people listening. You could break a new artist or move a new record or jump-start a new trend. The vampire hours were a tough adjustment, but I began to develop a following.

I stayed on the overnight shift for about six months. It's a great time to be on the air. In New York especially, you can be relaxed and more like yourself than you can during any other shift. You're not performing for your listeners, you're just hanging out with them.

During the week of Valentine's Day, 1985, I began a weeklong audition to join the station's morning program, along with the station's regular morning deejays, Richard Neer and Lisa Glasberg. The idea was for me to inject a little humor into the broadcast, which the station brass thought might help us compete with Howard Stern over at K-ROCK. It was a good idea and a miscalculation, all at the same time, because the only way to really compete with Howard was to stay out of his way. I remember it was Valentine's Day because we did a remote broadcast from Heartbreak, a club on Varick Street in Greenwich Village. The place was decked out with pink hearts. The Del Fuegos were there, performing live, which is always an interesting thing when it's seven o'clock in the morning. Somehow, live music never seems as loud as it does in the early hours of the morning, played in a club that would be otherwise empty.

I took the stage and told a couple jokes. I tried to make it like I wasn't performing, like I was just talking. I don't know if it was me or the Del Fuegos, but we had that place jumping, which meant my "audition" was going well. It went so well the general manager offered me the job, and I started the very next week. At first, I missed the music, but I didn't miss the late-night hours. And, we were up against Howard Stern, so this was another tough adjustment. Our station broadcast at 102.7 on the FM airwaves, and Stern was at 92.3, and we were as far apart in the ratings as we were on the dial.

For several weeks, our ratings were so dismal there was talk around the station that we were going to be fired. At first, we thought it was just talk, but then the general manager, Mike Kakyonias, called us in to tell us our days were numbered. We were just getting started, and already our days were numbered. This created a less-than-ideal environment for the three of us to relax and let our personalities shine through on the air. Instead we were constantly looking over our shoulders, wondering if each bit was being so closely scrutinized by station management that it couldn't possibly be deemed funny.

Sometimes, something struck us as funny but we were unable to let our listeners in on the joke, like the time Mick Jagger's longtime girlfriend Jerry Hall came to our studio. I remember thinking how remarkable this woman looked, so early in the morning. She had on a real put-together outfit, and she looked absolutely sensational—and completely out of place in our studio. The three of us were dressed like slugs, and here was Jerry Hall, looking like a page out of *Cosmo*. There was a real aura about her, but then as she spoke I looked down at her shoes and noticed she had enormous feet, and I had to bite my lip to keep from laughing. I was too much of a gentleman to point them out on the air.

Other times, we were funny when we didn't mean to be, like the time Tom Hanks came by to promote the movie *Big*. We played a game called "Rock 'n' Roll Jeopardy!" which was fairly self-explanatory. We asked Tom to tell the listeners at home what prizes they were playing for, and he put on a voice like one of those game show announcers.

I said, "Tom Hanks, tell them what they'll win!"

And he said, "Mark, they're playing for a WNEW alarm clock." Then he paused and said, "What a jive gift!"

We all laughed. It was a silly, off-the-wall thing to say, and it caught us by surprise. But our promotions director didn't think it was so funny. She thought we were making fun of the prize she had arranged for us to give away, so we took a little heat. We were always taking heat. Jay Leno came up to the station one morning to promote an area appearance, and before he arrived I played a tape from his show the night before. It never occurred to me that Jay didn't mean for us to use this tape, but I was called in to the music director's office at seven o'clock that morning. Jay was there. He said, "Where did you get that tape?"

I said, "Your agent sent it over."

He said, "No, he didn't."

Turns out it was the agent of the club Jay was appearing at. The guy was sending us tapes, hoping to boost advance ticket sales. After that, we weren't able to use taped performances. What worked best, really, was just the three of us being ourselves, not trying too hard. Typically, we'd try to find humor in everyday situations, tied in some way to whatever else was going on in the world. When the Mets were in the 1986 World Series against the Boston Red Sox, we called a bunch of different establishments in the Boston area, trying to find some displaced Mets fans. We thought it would be fun to find a Met fan in hostile territory. We even called a guy who ran a New York–style deli in Boston, thinking for sure he'd be a Met fan, but he said, "Sorry, guys. I'm a Red Sox fan."

We drew just a fraction of Howard Stern's audience, and finally my boss said he had to make a change. I understood that, although it wasn't our fault that we couldn't make a dent in Howard Stern's ratings. It was just a miscalculation. At just that moment in New York radio, no one could have taken on Howard Stern.

Once you've worked in New York you're not likely to consider a step-down to a smaller market until you're desperate. I was anxious, but I was far from desperate. I'd been doing some commercials. I had an agent who kept sending me on auditions, and I kept getting hired. I did a spot for Federal Express. I did a beer ad for Miller Lite. I did an Eastern Airlines commercial. At one point,

I even had a McDonald's commercial running at the same time as a Burger King commercial. The commercials paid good money, so I wasn't hurting financially, but the work could be spotty, and I had to think that one of the reasons I was booking so many of them was because I didn't really need the work.

I was out of a job, but I wasn't really out of work. I was also doing some television spots, too, just before I was let go at WNEW, and some of that work was ongoing. My most visible gig was on HBO, as one of four fill-in hosts who helped to bridge the time between movies. I interviewed Harvey Fierstein for one of these HBO segments, which I believe was my first "celebrity" interview.

The week I was fired, I did a commercial for Campbell's Soup, and I left that shoot to go out looking for full-time work. For a while, I thought I'd land a spot on K-ROCK in the afternoon, as a kind of bookend to Howard Stern in the morning. That was my dream job, but it never materialized. I did manage to get an interview for a veejay job at VH1, MTV's mellower sister channel, but that wasn't a dream job. That was just a job.

Into this strange career limbo came an unlikely opportunity. I gave an interview to the New York *Daily News*, about life after WNEW, and when the article appeared there were pictures of me and my former WNEW colleagues. It was a very positive piece. The producers at the new morning show at CBS read the article and thought I might be a good fit. Before the week was out, I had an audition at a soundstage in Manhattan. Bob Saget was there. I knew Bob from a television show I used to do called *Comedy Tonight*. I was the sidekick. The show featured up-and-coming comics. Bob was one of our guests. He was about to catch a break of his own with *Full House*, but for now he was banking on morning television to help make his name. He'd been hired to tell jokes and lighten the mood for a new CBS morning show that was now apparently also considering hiring me.

Then as now, there was a lot of controversy over at CBS regarding the morning show format. For many years, the network had been beaten badly in the mornings by its competitors, so now CBS was revamping, retooling, and recasting a new show to fill the time slot. Throughout the 1960s and 1970s, the network had ceded the morning news battleground to ABC and NBC, choosing instead to fill the time with an hour of *Captain Kangaroo* and an hour of straight news. In 1982, when *Captain Kangaroo* was finally cancelled, the network moved to a two-hour morning show format, but with disappointing results. A revolving door of anchors, including Bill Kurtis, Diane Sawyer, Phyllis George, and Maria Shriver, couldn't seem to win viewers over from the more established *Today* and *Good Morning America* broadcasts.

And so, the network went at it again, this time

pulling the two-hour morning show slot from the news division and handing it over to the entertainment division, a move seen by some in-house news wonks as a kind of sacrilege. The move was not unprecedented. Over at ABC, *Good Morning America* was produced by the network's entertainment division. At NBC, the *Today* show was in the hands of the news division. But at CBS, where news had helped to put and keep the network on the map, it was a seismic shift.

That's where I came in. I met with a guy named Bob Shanks, the executive producer of the new morning program, which was to be called *The Morning Program.* I went in to see Bob at CBS headquarters on 52nd Street—"Black Rock," to CBS staffers. The phone kept ringing as we talked, but Bob let it ring. He asked me a series of casual questions. The Mets had just won the 1986 World Series, so he asked me a couple questions about baseball. He asked me where I was born. He asked me about the weather. He was sizing me up, trying to see if I could think quickly and talk comfortably about a variety of different subjects. He must have seen something he liked, because after a while he sent me out to the waiting room to get my audition tape. When I got back, he said, "How do you feel about doing the weather?"

I didn't know the first thing about being a weatherman.

Bob said, "Don't worry, we'll get you a meteorologist."

So I said, "Fine." He could have asked me how I felt about being ten feet tall.

As I left his office, Bob said, "Do me a favor. Don't tell anyone about this meeting." At the time, news leaks about the CBS morning show experiment and the rift between the news and entertainment divisions were occupying a good deal of attention in the media, and I guess Bob wanted to avoid any scrutiny until he'd made all his personnel decisions.

I said, "Of course not." Then I left and told everyone I knew.

Two days later, I was on a CBS soundstage for my audition. I did a fake weathercast, with no map behind me. I said, "It's raining in Chicago. That must be the tears of the Cub fans coming down again."

Everyone laughed, and I left the studio to hand-shakes and congratulations. One of my well-wishers was the actress Mariette Hartley, fresh off those Pola-roid commercials with James Garner, who was due to be the show's cohost. Mariette held out her hand and said, "Welcome to the show." I shook it and thought, I think I got this job.

BIRC

Looks Like We're in for Nasty Weather

always told my speech therapist Tommi Ann I'd follow her anywhere, and after three or four weeks at Lucerne I did just that. She moved to a rehabilitation facility right across the street from the hospital. For Tommi Ann, it was a good career move. For me, it was a lifesaver.

Together, we went to a rehab facility called the Brain Injury Recovery Center—or BIRC for short. I've since learned that there are BIRC centers located all over the country, but back then I wasn't thinking so much about its national reputation. I was just thinking about Tommi Ann.

One of the reasons I placed so much faith in the hands of Tommi Ann, I think, was because as a speech therapist, she was, I believed, the key to my full recovery. My concerns going forward were different than the concerns of most patients. In my mind at least, Tommi Ann's focus was in my area of greatest, most immediate need. Because of this, I had no choice but to place her in such a fundamental role, and she fit right into it.

Forget for a moment Tommi Ann's particular area of expertise, and consider only her training and her role as the de facto coordinator of my rehabilitation. You'd think the essential follow-up care and recovery treatment for me would be under the guidance of a neurologist or a neurosurgeon, someone like Dr. Medary or Dr. Bagnoli who had supervised my care at the outset. The parallels in other areas of medicine are apparent. If you have a heart attack, your case is managed by a cardiologist. If you have cancer, there's an oncologist or some other doctor specializing in your particular form of cancer. If you suffer from depression and have been hospitalized as a result, you'll likely be in the supervisory care of a psychiatrist. But there was no such specialist or primary care physician to track my recovery. I saw Dr. Medary three more times after I left Sand Lake, for follow-ups and an MRI, most recently in December 2006. Dr. Bagnoli checked in on me when I first arrived at Lucerne, before he essentially handed me off to the hospital's therapists. As far as the neurological effects of my stroke were concerned, and any related medical issues, I was consigned to the care of my regular doctor—a wonderful man named Dr. John Hirt, who had a generalist's experience as well as some personal experience in this area, which meant that Denise and I were left to cobble together a treatment plan by ourselves, and this in turn meant we looked to Tommi Ann to become a kind of point person for my recovery.

There's no question that in my case my reliance on Tommi Ann was also due to the fact that she was a speech therapist, and that I made my living with my voice. It was a natural fit. Unlike most stroke patients, I was more concerned with how I sounded than how I looked or how I moved from here to there. The other patients I met at Sand Lake, Lucerne, and BIRC were mostly worried about walking and driving, getting around on their own, and doing for themselves. Me, I just wanted to talk. Like I used to. On the radio. On television. For my entire adult life, people knew me as a smooth-talking, quick-witted guy. It wasn't just my job, it was my personality. It was how I looked out at the world. I was always the one with the witty retort, the glib reply, the easy comeback. The expression you hear to describe people like me is that we think fast on our feet, although in my experience it had nothing to do with my feet. It was all about the mind, the sense of humor, the ability to set people at ease, the soothing voice.

My thinking was, Let me at least get my voice back to where it was, and I can worry about all those other moving parts later. In my case I wouldn't necessarily be able to walk like I did, or move the right side of my body with any kind of ease or grace, but viewers at home would never notice. From the neck up, sitting behind an anchor desk, I'd be the old me.

At first, I thought I'd be back to work after just a couple months. It didn't matter to me that I couldn't hold a pencil with my right hand, or that I was still a long way from being able to have a catch with one of my boys. All I needed to be able to do was sit at the anchor chair and read the news, and all I needed for that was my voice. Everything else would just fall into place after that. Or maybe it wouldn't, but I told myself I'd be okay with that, as long as I was able to work. Outside of work, at least I'd be able to crack a joke, or draw people out in conversation. Already, in just a few weeks, I'd made great gains in speech therapy, and there was no reason to think my progress wouldn't continue at this rate. I didn't know at the time that stroke patients make their most profound gains during the first three to six months of recovery. I was not yet aware that conventional rehab wisdom held that if you didn't get back certain abilities within a year following your stroke, you weren't likely to get them back at all. But in my travels I've talked to many stroke survivors. Almost everyone who was doing well said conventional stroke rehab reasoning didn't apply to them. They've seen, and continue to see gains, years after having a stroke. Almost everyone who was struggling pointed to the old way of thinking as the main reason they could never get past this or that hurdle.

Indeed, I was so confident of my continued rapid recovery that I actually mapped out my return to WKMG with Skip Valet and Henry Maldonado, thinking it would only be a matter of time before I could deliver the news without any slurring or impairment—but, alas, this turned out to be wishful thinking on my part. Skip and Henry turned out to be far more supportive of me and my recovery than I had any right to expect. They were model employers and wonderful friends. Tellingly, they were frequent visitors to my hospital bedside, and they continued to visit me at home. They were there for me in every conceivable way—and in some inconceivable ways, too. When I was finally able to get around on my own, they invited me out to dinner and to other events around town. They couldn't have been more patient or compassionate or otherwise considerate—although I knew full well they couldn't hold my job open for me indefinitely. They could keep me on the payroll. They could keep me up to date with my health insurance. But once it became clear that I wasn't able to *hurry back*, the way Skip had at first urged, they needed to put someone else in my morning and noon anchor chair. That was just business.

Back then, I was still thinking I'd go back to that job, and that the new person they were hiring would only keep that anchor chair warm for me. My thinking would change, over time, but there was a long road still ahead.

One of our biggest worries during this time was how much all this hospital care and outpatient therapy was going to cost. Our health insurance company paid for most of my hospitalization and rehab. It was up to us to meet our deductible. Insurance covered basic treatment and therapy, but Denise and I were always on the lookout for more innovative treatments and more progressive kinds of therapy. You can be sure that if I didn't seek out a particular treatment or therapy, the health insurance company wouldn't have mentioned it, even if it had been proven effective in similar cases. That's the nature of the patient-insurer relationship. It's not necessarily adversarial, but I wouldn't call it patient-friendly either. Yes, the insurance company wants the patient to recover quickly, but not because they're big-hearted and well-meaning. No, they want patients who require little or no hospitalization or therapy or aftercare, while the patient is usually pulling the relationship in the opposite direction, seeking the best possible treatment for at least as long as his condition requires it, even if his need outlasts his benefits.

Denise did a wonderful job shielding me from any health insurance concerns. It was her job to worry, she said, and mine to get better, although in truth there was really nothing to worry about. Denise handled all the paperwork, and ran interference for me—another key. You really do need a healthy, available, committed person to help guide you through the forms and regulations confronting hospital and long-term care patients today, when the best interests of the patient often collide with the bottom-line interests of health insurance companies. That said, I don't mean to give the impression that my own insurance company didn't come through for me. It did, in a big way. I happened to have a strong, far-reaching plan, with Aetna, and they really did right by me and my family during this ordeal, but I didn't have to look too far up and down the hallways at Sand Lake or Lucerne to see stroke victims being let out the door when their coverage dried up.

I was fortunate. Others, less so. I can't tell you how many times I saw a patient leave Lucerne before he or she was ready, simply because his or her insurance ran out. They couldn't walk on their own or take care of their basic needs. It was a heartbreaking, frustrating thing to see—and it happens all the time.

In my own case, fortunate or not, it was an endless chore for Denise to keep track of all the bills and forms, and to obtain the necessary approvals and referrals—leaving me with a clear head to focus on my rehabilitation and recovery. She never complained, or asked me to share the burden. Like I said before, she was my rock, and this was just one example of how she stood by me and stepped up during my recovery. Her thinking was, she could have fallen apart or held it together, and since I was the one whose body was quite literally falling apart it fell to her to help put me back together again. I was Humpty Dumpty; she was All the King's Horses and All the King's Men. She said she had no choice but to be strong and to stay on top of things for both of us, and one of the ways she did this was to slog through all this insurance stuff.

At one point, about a year after my stroke, when I was

finally driving and shaving and nearly back to my old self, I asked Denise if she could put a price tag on my hospital and rehab care. We were just talking, and it seemed like this would be a good piece of information for me to have. By this point, I was speaking and making public appearances on behalf of the National Stroke Association and the American Stroke Association, and I thought knowing the number would be useful. Denise responded that I didn't want to know the number, but I assured her that I did, so she went back through her files and took out a calculator and went at it. About an hour or so later, she called me in to show me the final total, and I took one look and nearly had another stroke: $250,000, and counting.

Understand, these weren't our out-of-pocket costs. This was the grand total—every co-payment we made, every bill that was paid by Aetna on our behalf, plus the cost of every pill I ingested or therapeutic device I needed to wear or piece of equipment I needed to purchase as part of my rehabilitation. It doesn't include the fees that were waived or reduced because they exceeded whatever Aetna deemed usual and customary in that area—just the monies that were actually paid to cover my medications, consultations, tests, treatments, and hospital costs. That's a big number, wouldn't you agree? And yet it's relatively small when you stand it alongside a comparable figure for cardiac patients, especially those who undergo bypass surgery, or cancer patients, especially those who sign on for chemotherapy or radiation treatments.

Again, the health insurance costs really weren't an issue for me—in part, because I had Denise riding herd over the situation, and also because I had an excellent health plan. I'm acutely aware that cost is very often an issue for other stroke patients and their families, a big issue, but I don't think I was even aware of any billing worries or insurance snafus, back when I was ramping down at Lucerne and ramping up at BIRC. I've since learned there were a few small glitches Denise had to get past, but she pretty much left me alone to do my thing. She had it covered.

Thanksgiving came and went before I left Lucerne, and I mention it here for the picture it paints of my loving wife and the family life she managed to nurture and sustain during my hospital stay. This, too, was key, because the rest of your life doesn't need to be put on pause simply because your body has momentarily given out. Denise was determined to put out our usual holiday feast at our home, complete with all the relatives and trimmings. She wasn't about to let a little thing like my massive stroke spoil a holiday tradition for our kids, so she set about her usual preparations. She cooked up a storm. She filled the house with friends and family. And then, after everyone was well-fed, and drunk on good cheer (and good pie!), she snuck out to Lucerne to see me. She brought a small plate of turkey and stuffing and whatever else she thought I might like. And then we sat together quietly, as Denise filled me in on what I'd missed at home.

I'd missed a lot, I knew. And I would miss a lot more.

Not just Thanksgiving, but more than a month of the business-as-usual stuff that makes up a family. Our boys were still so young that every day was filled with all kinds of discoveries, and I'd missed a bunch of milestone moments. And forget the milestones—I'd missed a bunch of those all-important, everyday moments as well. Reading to them at night. Going to museums. Teaching them to swim. I mean, my little guys were only going to be this age once. They were at that time in their development where you feel like if you blink you might miss something, and here I'd done a lot of blinking. And it wasn't just the boys. Denise's daughter, Jenna, was growing up faster than her mother and I could fathom, so even just a few weeks apart from her was a lot. And my own daughter, Maya, lived with her mother in New York, and I hated the way my time in the hospital kept me from what I'd already come to regard as our too-infrequent visits. It sometimes felt like the moving sidewalk of my life just kept rolling along without me, and I was stuck on the curb until I could jump back on.

I might have been feeling stuck, a little bit, but at the same time I'd made enormous progress in a fairly short stretch of time. Here is what I couldn't do when I entered Lucerne, about a week after my stroke: walk on my own power, hold a book steady enough to read, go to the bathroom, feed myself, put my thoughts into words without extreme effort, talk without sounding like a Saturday morning cartoon, lift my right arm above my head.

Here is what I could do when I left Lucerne, over three

weeks later: roam the hallways without the aid of a walker, turn the pages of *The New York Times*, shower, dial a number on my cell phone, open a car door, eat with a fork, make love with my wife.

Progress? You better believe it. I went from not being able to recognize the man I was in the man I had become, to believing I might return in full to the man I was before stroke. My entire outlook had changed—and I credit Tommi Ann and Walter and my ever-changing team of good-hearted therapists for creating such a positive, hopeful, energetic environment. I always believed I would make a complete recovery. Now, whatever lingering doubts I might have had were falling away. Now there would be no stopping me.

My biggest concern upon leaving Lucerne was going home. For the longest time, this had been the carrot-on-a-stick I held out for myself during those grueling physical therapy sessions with Walter. I'd tell myself I just had to do one more set, one more repetition, one more minute, whatever it happened to be, and I'd be that much closer to the day I could go home. It was all I really thought about, all I really wanted, and then it was upon me.

Remember, I'd already been back home on that eventful day pass, so it's not like I was covering entirely new ground, but it was a big deal just the same. It wasn't so much a concern about being home and returning to my familiar spaces and routines. That part was welcome. It was about fitting myself back in to our lives. That's where it would get hard. I didn't know what my role would be—what it *could* be, even. What kind of dad could I be to my children, if I couldn't walk and talk and jump and play with them the way I always had? Would Denise have to drop what she was doing to take care of me, instead of taking care of the kids? Would I be such a drain on the wellspring of resources in our family that the love and laughter that had stamped our household for as long as I could remember might suddenly disappear? And what about in the bedroom? Yes, I know Denise and I had already dipped our toe in these waters, but when you're left to your own thoughts on the rehab unit all day your mind comes up with all kinds of questions, and not a whole lot of answers.

There was one giant question mark after another looming over my move back home, and Denise and I decided that the best way to answer those daunting open questions was to just meet them head-on. I tried to talk to her about some of these things, but she said there was nothing to talk about—not in a dismissive way, but in a helpful, reassuring way. She said everything would be just fine, so of course I believed her. The thing to do, she said, was to jump right back in to how our lives used to be, in whatever ways possible. Anyway, that was our plan, and so on the first Monday after I was home I headed off to BIRC like I had a job to do. I made rehabilitation my career, my focus, my priority. Denise got Jenna off to school, packed the boys in the car, and drove me and the boys the twenty or so miles to BIRC, where my therapists went to work on me.

My days at BIRC were much the same as they had been

at Lucerne, except I was assigned a new physical therapist. Walter would arrive at BIRC a short time later, and pick up where he left off, but in the beginning I worked with a couple different therapists. My first physical therapist at BIRC was named Rod Olson. He was in charge of the entire facility, as well as being the chief physical therapist. Rod, I learned, was from a small town in Michigan. As a young man, he worked summers at the printing mill where his father also worked. He was a second baseman as a kid, so we immediately struck up a friendship and talked baseball and physical therapy. I was still using a walker when I started at BIRC, and one of the first tasks Rod set out for me was a stepping exercise. He worked it out on his computer. He had me stepping up and down off a series of blocks he'd laid out on the floor. I had to step over a block, stop on a block, step down from a block. Over and over. Soon, we progressed to going up stairs. He worked a lot on my balance, because the stroke had really done a number on my balance. I tended to fall over quite easily. I didn't lose strength, but I did lose balance, so Rod had me working with one of those big exercise balls, to help develop my core.

The biggest change to my days once I started at BIRC was that I began doing occupational therapy as well. Occupational therapy focuses on your writing, your driving, your thinking. Essentially, all the simple tasks you need to complete without thinking about them in order to get through your day come under the heading of occupational therapy. There had been some basic occupational therapy sessions at

Lucerne, certain specific tasks and objectives that had been layered into the other therapy I was doing there, but I had yet to work with an occupational therapist in any kind of orchestrated, sustained way.

My first few OT sessions were devoted mainly to intelligence-type tests. The therapist would hold up an image and I would have to describe what I saw. It wasn't a Roschach test, but it was the same type of thing. I'd have to find patterns or images inside the shapes. Or, I'd have to look at three similar pictures and identify the difference in one of them. It was like being on a game show.

That's an easy laugh line, but it's also the truth. The way they had these sessions set up, it really did feel like a game show. I was a guest on *Hollywood Squares*, back when John Davidson was the host. The questions and tasks my therapists set out for me seemed a lot like the questions and tasks the *Hollywood Squares* producers came up with when I appeared early on in my run at CBS. I was told it was the first time they had a weatherman on the panel. I was in the bottom right-hand square, all the way in the corner. Joan Rivers was the center square. The prop department set it up so there was a window in my square, and whenever they called on me for a question they made it rain or snow or sleet. It was funny. All my questions were weather-related. They gave you a list of suggested responses, but you were free to come up with your own improvised answer. We taped five shows Saturday and five shows Sunday. The only difference between these OT sessions and my *Hollywood Squares* experience, really, was that this time out I didn't have to worry about making an audience laugh.

To be honest, I didn't take my OT sessions all that seriously at first. I thought, I don't need to do this. I thought, It's taking time away from my speech therapy and my physical therapy. Whatever question they threw at me, I just gave any answer, without even thinking about it, only what I didn't know was that there was no *right* answer. Whatever I said, for whatever reason, that was the right answer. It was the right answer simply because it was the answer I gave, and was therefore the true indication of what I was thinking and feeling.

Later on, they had me doing all kinds of useful, relevant exercises that would help me do things like open a jar, button my shirt, or write with my right hand. Absolutely, the OT work I did with my therapists turned out to be enormously helpful. But for the first week or so, I resisted it. In one of the tests, there were pictures of four different squares. They were mostly alike, with a few subtle differences. One of the squares might have had a different pattern to it. Another was slightly larger than the other three. I was supposed to identify which square was different and explain why it was different. This was in the beginning, so I just pointed to a square, and as a result they thought I was worse off than I really was. They thought I couldn't recognize the subtle differences, and that the stroke had done some more serious damage to the part of my brain that pays attention to things like subtle differences.

Tommi Ann knew the score. My therapists would compare notes and monitor my progress in these other areas, and she knew right away I wasn't trying my hardest on these tests. By this point Tommi Ann knew me well enough to know my answers were being tossed off without a thought, so she impressed on me that I was only hurting myself by failing to take this stuff seriously. I hadn't thought about it in just this way, but she was right. She said it undermined what we were accomplishing in speech therapy, and the strides I was making in physical therapy. She was right about this, too.

Eventually, I got it. Eventually, I started to trust that these good people knew what they were doing. I believe I started out thinking this was something I was doing for them, for the therapists, instead of something I was doing for me, and once I got that my whole attitude changed. Once again, I had Tommi Ann to thank for setting me straight—because nothing was more important. After all, this was now my job, and I owed it to myself and my family to give it my best effort in every aspect. I told myself I had no choice.

After "work" each day, I returned home to my loving and supportive family, and tried to fit myself back into how we were before my stroke. I'd walk in the door and hear the sounds of *Little Bear* or *Maisy* coming from the television— two of the boys' favorites at the time. It was welcome background noise, because there was a time just a few short months earlier when I couldn't have told you what my boys were watching on television. I liked that I was plugged back in to our daily lives—although, of course, I wasn't plugged all the way back in. When I first got home, I couldn't do a lot as far as playing went with the boys. They didn't seem to mind. They were just glad daddy was home. As time went on and I got stronger and stronger, the fun and games with them increased. I wasn't sure there was a place for me at first. I couldn't get down on all fours and roughhouse with the boys the way I used to, and I couldn't shoot hoops in the driveway or throw a football around. I couldn't make dinner or help with the dishes. I couldn't even drive the kids to school, or to their friends' houses to play. I was determined to get life back to the way it was, and determined to once again be the man I once was, but mostly I was an observer. I was participating and not participating, all at once. I was trying to be helpful around the house, but in truth I knew I was not as much help as I used to be. All I could do, really, was stay out of the way and try to take care of myself and my own basic needs, while Denise scrambled to take care of the house and the kids.

I don't mean to sound like I was despondent over this situation, because that certainly wasn't the case. I'm generally a happy-go-lucky, positive person. Things tend to roll off of me, even big things like recovering from my stroke. Me feeling like there was no place for me at home was entirely in my head. Certainly there was a place for me, it's just that it wasn't the same place as before. A big part of me was overjoyed to be out of the hospital, surrounded by my family and warmed by the comforts of hearth and home. But there were very definitely some adjustments.

I considered my relationship with Denise. If I was truly her partner, I thought, then poor Denise was getting the raw end of the deal. Over time, I took on more and more responsibilities around the house, as my recovery allowed. I could fix meals for the kids, change diapers, and help the boys get ready for school. I could help Denise coordinate everyone's after-school activities. Gradually, I allowed myself to think I was back in the mix, even before I was fully ready to resume a full-throttled parenting role.

Some days, I'd return home from a difficult session at BIRC and shut myself in my den for an hour or two before dinner. I used the time to read over some of the mail that had come in, and to return some of the phone calls I received during the day. These calls were always a great lift. I talked to my dad, and my siblings. I talked to old friends at CBS, and new friends at WKMG. I heard from long-lost friends. I remember one such call from my friend Tony Bennett that left me soaring. Tony and I had met a long time ago at the Rainbow Room in New York City. He was a legend back then, but not the legend he is today. It was a couple years before the career resurgence he enjoyed in the 1990s, when he worked with artists like Elvis Costello and k.d. lang, and appeared on MTV's *Unplugged* before a new generation of fans.

It was a special thrill to meet him, and I told Tony as much when I had a chance to interview him for CBS.

We got along great, and over the years developed a fine friendship. He told me once I was like a contemporary Ed Sullivan. I took it as high praise. He paid me another great compliment a short time later when he launched a show on A&E called *Live by Request*. The idea of the show was to take call-in requests from viewers, almost like a radio show. The callers would share with the audience their particular memories of a particular song—where they first heard it, who they were with when they first heard it, what they were doing at the time, and what it all meant to them. Then Tony would sing the song. It was Tony's concept, and he was the perfect guy to bring it off, but he called me one day and said he needed a host. He said the format required an emcee-type person to tie everything together, and he thought I'd be just right for it, because of my affinity for the music and my ability to interview all kinds of people and make them feel comfortable.

I was flattered, but the network was something less than enthusiastic about the idea. They wanted a woman to do the honors, because the first show was to be on Valentine's Day 1996, and A&E liked the dynamics of a man and a woman working out in front on this, but Tony wanted me. Three times they asked him to reconsider, and three times he gave them my name.

In the end, Tony got what he wanted, but the producers of the show had never heard of me so they had no idea what they were getting. They wanted to script the entire show. They thought that was the best way to control the content.

I suggested they script only the intros and the outros, and leave the questions to Tony and the caller open-ended. I remembered that lesson I learned from my floor manager, about asking what I wanted to know, back when I did my first celebrity network interview. I said, "Live television, I'm used to. Live, I can do." Reluctantly, the producers agreed to let me wing it, and the show ended up winning an Emmy and running for seven years, but I wouldn't have gotten the gig if it hadn't been for Tony. He put his foot down to get me that job—not only as a kindness, but also because he thought I'd bring a nice spin to the project. He's a true, true friend. He called Denise as soon as he heard about my stroke, and he followed up with phone calls to see how I was doing.

One day soon after I returned home, Tony called just to chat. He marveled at how good I sounded, how strong. He was thrilled for me that I was finally out of the hospital, and well along on my uphill climb toward recovery. He said he thought I'd be back on television in no time flat. He knew what it was to work in front of a television camera and a microphone. He knew how important my voice was to me.

Then he got a little wistful and said, "Everyone I've ever known who had a stroke went away." He was silent for a while, and then he said, "You're the only one who's ever come back."

Coming from Tony Bennett, that was praise indeed. You have to realize, Tony was older than me. He'd known dozens and dozens of people who had been felled by stroke.

Me, I'd known hardly anyone at all. So to hear him marvel at how well I was doing, and how I was the first person he knew to ever fight his way back from stroke, it was a wonderful thing indeed. If it was anybody else on the other end of the phone, I might have broken out in song. Since it was Tony Bennett, I could only close my eyes and smile and thank him for the power of his thoughts and good wishes.

Those quiet few hours in my den at the end of each day were a great way for me to decompress and steel myself for the hard work of the next day. Sometimes, I grabbed those few hours later in the evening, after the kids were asleep, or in the early hours of the morning, before anyone else in the house was awake. During this time in my den, I found the Internet to be an excellent rehabilitation tool, although I had a hard time working the keyboard at first. There were times when my fingers felt like sausages, typing away on those tiny keys, but I managed. My right hand especially gave me some trouble as I struggled to type, but the chance to communicate with friends and family online and to seek out information and insights on stroke and related issues was extremely liberating.

A lot of stroke patients I talk to tell me how they feel shut-in and closed off from the rest of the world during the early stages of their recovery. Their normal routines have been upended by their condition, and a great many report feeling left behind by their circle of friends. They talk about how people are usually pretty good about coming by for a visit in the beginning, and how those visits start to thin as people return to their own lives and calendars, their own ups and downs. They talk about missing those all-important points of connection at work, and feeling like the world is passing them by. I had some of those same feelings, in varying degrees, and I tried to put a positive spin on things, but when I came up short the Internet was a great equalizer. It made it easier for me to keep in touch with friends and colleagues, and to feel plugged in to what was going on beyond my front door, so I spent a lot of time online. I'd always been big into e-mail, but in the first blush of recovery I think I spent more time online than ever before. I believe this carried a physical therapy benefit as well, because it forced me to use my fingertips to tap on the keyboard. I cheated a lot at first, using my left more than I should have, but my right hand got a good workout, too. Without really realizing it, I'd developed my own form of therapy, reconditioning the muscles in my right hand to respond to simple commands and perform simple tasks—while at the same time reaching out to a world I was eager to rejoin.

Very quickly, we fell into a new routine. I went to BIRC every day for three hours each morning. The drill was we'd get Jenna off to school, then Denise would pack me and the boys into our Toyota minivan and head out. It took us a while to get our act together each morning. I was still moving pretty slowly, so washing and shaving and dressing was a painstaking process. To complicate things, the rehab center wasn't exactly around the corner, so Denise had to find something to do with herself and the boys to keep from making the round-trip commute twice each day. It was the same trip she was used to making to Lucerne, but there she could visit in the evening when things were a little quieter at home, when we had some help. My BIRC sessions were in the heart of the day.

Leave it to my wife to give new meaning to the term "multitasking." She discovered a great, full-service gym not too far from the rehab center, where they had a day care program for Miles and Griffin. So Denise started going to the gym every day, for three hours, and before she knew it she was in the best shape of her life. We used to joke that we could market our own exercise program on the back of our ordeal. All you have to do is have your partner suffer a major stroke, and force yourself to fill the time during his or her therapy by going to the gym.

Piece of cake, right?

In all seriousness, those daily sessions at the gym were a kind of salvation for Denise. She looked up one morning and realized she was growing more powerful and energized and confident each day. And, she told me later, she came to look forward to those three-hour gym sessions as a pocket of calm in her busy days—the "eye" in the storm our lives had become. Most important, I think, was that she was doing something for herself, at the same time she was doing something for me and our family.

This went on for about three months, and in that time I made enormous gains as well. I was also stronger, and more confident. I also came to look forward to my sessions at

BIRC, the same way a marathon runner logs those all-important training miles. I slipped into a kind of zone. I was focused, determined, committed to getting back to how I was. I knew it would be a series of small steps, but I knew that each step was taking me closer to my goal and that each was more important than the one that preceded it. I was also doing something for myself, at the same time I was doing something for Denise and our family. The more I was able to do for myself, the more my limitations seemed to get to me. I hated that I couldn't drive. This was an issue in our household, because I relied exclusively on Denise to get around, and there were so many other things she could be doing. Plus, I felt like I was such a burden, to have to be ferried around like that. Denise never minded, of course, but I felt like a burden just the same.

I thought, Driving shouldn't be so hard, so I went to Dr. Hirt to discuss it. In my mind it was a small thing, but I needed a doctor's approval in order to prove to the Motor Vehicle Department and to my automobile insurance carrier that I was fit to resume driving. More than that, I needed to know I wasn't about to put myself, my passengers, or anyone else in danger by being back on the road. We had three cars: the Toyota minivan, a BMW convertible, and a 1987 Porsche. Denise usually drove the Toyota, but since my stroke she was trying to put some miles on our other cars as well, just to keep them thrumming. Of all the things we had to worry about, this was one of the things we worried

about. Already, I'd practiced pulling in and out of our driveway in my Porsche, using my right hand to work the stick
shift. The car had been one of my favorite toys, and it had
been in the garage for the longest time. I longed to take it
out into the bright Florida sunshine. It felt like an exten-
sion of my own confinement—because I was feeling as
cooped up as my car. I was ready to step on the gas.

Dr. Hirt was sympathetic to my position. His own wife
had suffered a stroke many years before mine. He knew full
well what it meant to be kept from the simple, daily tasks
we almost take for granted—like driving. I'd been working
for several weeks by this point with an occupational therapist at BIRC named Suzy Rentz, whose main focus was on
getting me to do and think for myself. In her assessment,
this included driving a car. It wasn't her primary objective
to get me back behind the wheel, but it was one of her many
goals for me. To this end, she had me doing all kinds of different exercises. Most of them had nothing at all to do with
driving, or hand-eye coordination, or any of the other skills
I thought it was important for me to relearn. In one, she had
me doing a kind of word search with numbers. She gave me
a grid, marked with random numbers, and I'd have to find a
specific sequence or pattern in the grid. She'd say, "Okay,
Mark, now show me 9-8-7-5-6-1-3-1-3-6-4-5-9," and I'd
frantically search the grid while she ran a stopwatch and
recorded my time. I struggled with these number searches
at first. I took a bunch of them home with me, which I was

supposed to complete in under an hour. It took me about four hours that first time. I completed them, so there was accomplishment in that, but I knew I had to work at it.

I didn't realize it at the time, but these exercises were training the left side of my brain, so while Denise was off at the gym, gaining fitness and strength in her own workout, and reenergizing herself for the rest of the day, I was in rehab doing workouts of my own. I worked so long and hard on this stuff, you'd think I had a six-pack of muscles up there inside my head.

There were also a whole bunch of counseling-type sessions that Suzy put me through. I didn't get the point of these at first, either. She'd ask me questions like, "What would you do if a stranger peeked through your window at home?" I answered in a very concrete way. I said I lived in a gated community, so it wasn't likely that someone would be peeking through our window unless it was someone I already knew. Suzy said this answer was unacceptable, and encouraged me to come up with another. This time I said I'd go get Denise or call the police—both practical responses, I thought.

Suzy put a lot of these kinds of questions and scenarios to me, and in response to each I'd say, "I'd go get Denise." Or, "I'd call the police." Of course, she wanted me to indicate a bit more self-reliance, and discover solutions to problems that I could handle myself, but I wasn't quite there in my thinking. It was emblematic. When I was confident in my ability to take care of myself and do for myself, Suzy said, my answers to these questions would reflect that. Until then, Denise would continue to take care of me.

Suzy also tested me on any number of first aid and emergency response–type scenarios. The thinking here, I guess, was that once I was able to offer an adequate response to these questions, once I was able to think quickly through a series of stressful situations, then I'd be ready to think about getting back behind the wheel and taking on some additional responsibilities with the kids at home.

I was a long way from the autonomy I now craved, but I was getting there.

LIFE BEFORE STROKE: *CBS*

*T*he *Morning Program* premiered on CBS on January 12, 1987. *Entertainment Tonight* came to our studio on West 57th Street to cover our debut. Mariette Hartley brought her golden retriever, Daisy, to the set. That should tell you right there that we were a little different than the other network morning shows. We had a studio audience—another big difference. We had stand-up comics. And we had a former stand-up comic-turned-radio-deejay-turned-weatherman to tell you what you could see for yourself if you just looked out the window.

We were a work-in-progress, to start. Nobody really told me what to do or say, only where to stand. I was basically on my own. For my very first weather segment,

I pointed to Mariette's dog and said, "It's cold outside, not like Daisy's favorite days, the dog days of summer." The audience groaned. My new CBS colleagues groaned. So I said, "Shoot me." They were right to groan, I guess, but I just laughed and reported the weather. The television critics also groaned. Howard Rosenberg of the *Los Angeles Times* said he would do two things if he was in charge of the network; he would scrap the format and the weatherman.

I thought, So much for auspicious beginnings.

It turned out Howard Rosenberg was right about one thing and wrong about another. The keen minds at CBS tinkered with the format and the talent lineup of the morning show so often during our first year it's a wonder we found any audience at all. They also decided to keep me around. Whenever there was a shake-up on the program, I managed to survive the shaking. The producers seemed to like my style—and, according to their research, so did the viewers.

One day I looked up and realized I had carved out a nice niche for myself. Along with my producer, Kevin Coffey, we reinvented the role of the morning show weatherperson. We took what Willard Scott had been doing for years on the *Today* show at NBC, and added our own spin to it. We started doing all kinds of stunts for the cameras. Some of them were harebrained. Some of them were dangerous. Some of them were exotic. And almost all of them were fun.

My CBS colleagues called me Smokey the Bear, because it fell to me to travel the country, visiting our affiliate stations where the ratings were low. Our job was to put out any fires of discontent before they spread. If station management was unhappy with the network fare that season, or if their local news ratings were lagging because our show was failing to attract an audience, I went and made nice. I was like an ambassador for the network. Network executives weren't about to go themselves to these good people, so they sent me and a camera crew instead. I'd usually come in the night before, have dinner with the affiliates, meet and greet some of the local viewers, and then get up at first light to do the weather from remote locations of interest. It became a real point of pride for these local stations, to host our happy crew and gain some national exposure.

Sometimes, we'd visit a different city every day. We'd start at one end of the country and work our way across: San Francisco, Tulsa, San Antonio, Miami, and Burlington, Vermont. It was a grueling schedule, but it was a blast. Kevin used to say it was the time of our lives, and he was right. It was. We were on the road more often than not. One month, somewhere in the middle of my fifteen-year run at CBS, I checked my calendar and realized I'd only slept in my own bed for three nights. Each time out, we came up with creative, interesting segments that took me to curious, out-of-the-way places our viewers wouldn't normally get a chance to see. Once there, I'd do four segments each morning, usually involving some stunt or other. I was never afraid to fall on my face. I was also a fast study. And, I was always game—and up for any challenge. You wouldn't think these traits were what you needed to succeed as a network weatherman, but my segments were never really about the weather. The weather was kind of an afterthought, like that Dylan line about not needing a weatherman to know which way the wind blows.

No, you don't. But you do need a weatherman, apparently, to know that the Finnish population of Hancock, Michigan, in the Upper Peninsula of Michigan, greatly appreciate it when you pronounce the word sauna as "sow-na" instead of "saw-na," and that the ore mines of the UP can get mighty cold and icky and wet, especially if you're huddled around down there for a while, waiting for your segment to begin.

I liked the small towns for the special attention we always received when we breezed in, and the chance to get to know the people and their traditions and to sample the homemade pies and cookies and other local recipes someone invariably brought down to the set. (A word of advice: morning show weatherman is not the best job if you're worried about your weight.) I liked the big towns because we often received a backstage pass to a side of these great cities and major tourist destinations that the rest of the world rarely got a chance to see. Kevin had me suiting up to take batting practice at spring training camps, or climbing into an F-15 fighter plane, or fly-fishing in Vermont. In a backhanded sort of way, I learned how the world worked, and how it didn't. I learned what was important to the American people, and what wasn't.

During my long stint at CBS, I covered almost every imaginable television event, including the Academy Awards, the Golden Globes, the Cannes Film Festival, the Grammy Awards, and the Country Music Association Awards. I also covered three Winter Olympics— in Albertville, Lillehammer, and Nagano, where I also served as anchor of CBS Sports' morning coverage. In my sideline role as a pop culture and entertainment reporter for the network, I interviewed hundreds of news makers, tastemakers, and decision makers, from Washington to Hollywood and points in between, including presidents Bill Clinton, George H. W. Bush, and Gerald Ford; Steven Spielberg, John Travolta, Sidney Poitier, Paul McCartney, Denzel Washington, Jim Carrey, Whoopi Goldberg, Julia Roberts, Tom Hanks, Madonna, and Joni Mitchell.

For the actual weather report, I relied on the talents and insights of a meteorologist named George Cullen. In the beginning, when fax machines were not yet ubiquitous, George would fax me some maps and I would look them over, and then we would talk on the phone and discuss the nation's weather. He'd tell me if it was raining here, or snowing there, or whatever. He was a nice man, content to work behind the scenes.

A lot of times, people would come to me and blame me for the lousy weather. They'd say, "I had an outdoor wedding, and it poured all day. Thanks a lot." It was always good-natured. In response I'd say, "How come you don't blame Dan Rather when he delivers bad news?"

In fifteen years at CBS, I worked with eight executive producers and four network news presidents, so I guess you could say television news is not the most stable environment. There's not a lot of job security. I also worked with more than a dozen on-air colleagues. Mariette Hartley, Rolland Smith, and Bob Saget made way for Harry Smith and former ABC stalwart Kathleen Sullivan. Kathleen eventually made way for Paula Zahn. Even my friend Harry, who has since returned to host the morning program, made way for yours truly, when I became coanchor in 1996, along with Jane Robelot, who signed on to replace Paula. After that it was my turn to enter the network's revolving door, when CBS hired former *Today* show host Bryant Gumbel and I decided to return to my weather post. Bryant was teamed with Jane Clayson. And, there was also a long list of newsreaders.

I liked my job a lot. It wasn't even a job I knew I wanted, but there it was. I never set out to be famous, but I didn't mind being recognized. It's not like I was some reviled public figure. My father used to tell me that one of the perks of my job was that people would tell you who you are. I'd meet someone in an airport, or on an elevator, or at the checkout line at the super-market, and they'd turn to me and say, "You're Mark McEwen."

And I would always thank them for pointing that out to me.

DRIVE

When They Said Sit Down I Stood Up

A big part of healing is psychological. I suppose I knew this on one level going in, but it's quite another thing to rediscover a sense of well-being and accomplishment and purpose that might have appeared lost to you. It's all tied in to how the rest of your body works, don't you think?

I know in my case that when I regained consciousness in that hospital bed at Sand Lake and began to puzzle together what had happened to me, I might have fallen so deep into despair that no amount of physical therapy could have helped me claw my way back out again. If I was a different type of person, I might not have even bothered to try. Consider the picture I took in: I couldn't move the right side of my body; I could barely move my left; I couldn't speak clearly enough to make myself understood. I was a complete mess. If ever there was a moment for me to feel down about myself or my situation, it was staring right back at me, but I didn't have it in me to quit or feel sorry for myself.

All I knew was to go straight ahead and confront my new circumstance.

I found my motivation where I could. At first it came from my personality. I wasn't a quitter, plain and simple. Going back to when I was a kid, I always had my fair share of drive and commitment. I saw something I wanted, and I reached for it. If I didn't grab it the first time around, I kept reaching. I got that perseverance from my parents, who taught it to us kids by their actions as much as by their words. By their example, we learned you could be anything you wanted to be. There were no limits but the limits we put on ourselves. After that, I think my present day motivation came from my own family. I wanted to get better, stronger for Denise and the kids. That was my focus.

There was one night, early on, when the space between my disabilities and my abilities seemed wider than I could ever hope to cross. We had a baby monitor in our bedroom, so we could listen to the boys after they went to sleep. One night not long after I came home from the hospital, before I started rehabbing at BIRC, one of the twins started to cry. The way it usually works with twins is when one of them starts something the other one is sure to follow. Denise and

I were both awakened by the crying, but I offered to take my turn and comfort the boys. Denise smiled and said she'd wait up for me. In her sleepy eyes I could see that she was glad to have me back, on the job, co-parenting. It had been hard on her, I knew, with me out of commission in the hospital all those weeks while she was at home with the kids, so I struggled out of bed and grabbed my walker and began the long, slow shuffle to the other side of the house, to the boys' bedroom. The kicker to the story is that it took me so long to get there that by the time I did the boys had fallen off to sleep, so I shuffled back to my bedroom. By the time I returned, Denise had drifted off back to sleep, too.

It would have been depressing if it hadn't been so funny, and as I tried to get back to sleep that night I couldn't shake the thought that I was a long way from my old self. At this pace, I thought, I couldn't be a father *or* a husband, but I determined to change that. BIRC would change that, I vowed. Tommi Ann would change that. Time would change that.

I would change that.

I finally did get around to driving. When Suzy was done putting me through my paces at BIRC, and I was given the green light by Dr. Hirt to get back behind the wheel, Denise demonstrated an enormous amount of confidence in me. She saw me headed out to the car that first afternoon and asked me to take the boys to the playground a mile or so from our house. She didn't even wait for me to get a couple practice runs under my belt. She just tossed me the keys and the kids and in this simple gesture told me she trusted me implicitly. It was a profound demonstration of love and faith, and I didn't take it lightly. I drove so slowly and methodically to the park you could have wheeled a Matchbox car down there and beaten me by a couple minutes, but it was a milestone accomplishment for me, and it came on the back of my wife's loving trust.

(If you're keeping score at home, I think I cried at the end of this moment, too.)

Some of my inspiration was external, and unintentional. I can still remember the first New Year's Eve I spent at home after I got out of the hospital. Like a lot of people, we turned on the television as midnight approached. We watched Dick Clark's *Rockin' New Year's Eve* celebration on ABC. Dick Clark was making his triumphant return to television, after suffering a stroke of his own. I looked on with a heavy heart and great empathy. For years, Dick Clark had been known as the ageless wonder of our popular culture. He looked as young and vital throughout the '70s, '80s, and '90s as he did when he was hosting *American Bandstand* in the '60s. Even into the first half of this decade, he looked great and continued to put a flourish to a remarkable career. But then stroke knocked him from the public eye, and now here he was, back on television. I was proud of him because he could have retreated into a private life and no one would have blamed him. Instead he was back at his post as if to say, "Here I am. Don't count me out just yet."

It occurred to me that I was probably one of the few

people who knew what Dick Clark was going through that night. I knew what it was to be sidelined by a sudden disability. I knew what it was to fight your way back to whole. I knew the pressure Dick was probably putting on himself, to get back on television as quickly as possible. And yet I also knew that it was too soon for me. I would go back to work on my terms, or not at all.

I'd always admired Dick Clark. He was an inspiration, and now that his life and legacy were also about stroke he was an inspiration in this area, too. I admired him even more that New Year's Eve, for bravely facing his demons and getting back to work. What I did for a living—what I *used* to do for a living, at least—was a little outside the curve for stroke patients. What was probably right and good and necessary for Dick Clark would not be right and good and necessary for me. There was no set calendar to mark my return, no other prominent stroke patients in my field against whom I could measure my progress. If I'd had a more typical desk job, I would have probably been back to work already. If Dick Clark had been an accountant, or a middle manager, or an advertising executive, he too would have been back at work and getting on with his life. But because we worked in television, beneath a harsh, unforgiving spotlight, we would be judged by a different standard.

I also drew inspiration from my therapists, only not in the ways they intended. Sure, I responded to their positive energy and enthusiasm, but it went beyond that. If one of them told me he or she hadn't seen a patient show such improvement in such a short stretch of time, I took that as a challenge to work harder still. I wasn't out to heal at a quicker rate than any of the other patients; I was out to get my life back, and soon.

All of these impulses were enough to get me headed in the right direction, but as I started making progress and talking to other stroke patients I discovered inspiration in a place I hadn't thought to look. This began to happen almost as soon as I left Lucerne and tried to ease back into the rest of my life. I found that it was enormously gratifying to speak to other people going through some of the same motions— and, on the flip side of the same deal, to share my experiences with them. I did this in an informal way at first, just swapping stories with other patients in rehab, or talking to friends and family members of some of the other patients on the unit, but very quickly these talks became more and more formal, as I started speaking to groups of patients and their primary caregivers. I found a new place to put all the energy and creativity that used to go into my work.

Let me tell you, it was a revitalizing thing, to be put through my paces with the eyes of the American stroke community upon me. While I was still at Lucerne, and to a greater extent while I was commuting to BIRC for my outpatient sessions there, I started to hear from doctors and therapists who suggested I could help others struggling through their own rehabilitations, or even help prevent strokes by promoting a heart-healthy lifestyle and other prevention measures. In the beginning, I didn't really understand why these people were looking to me on this, because I wasn't anywhere near where I wanted to be in my recovery. I wasn't any kind of role model. I wasn't completely healed or back to my old self. And I certainly wasn't any kind of authority on stroke. I was doing the best I could, that's all. I was making great gains, this was true, but there was a lot of hard work still ahead. And I still wasn't comfortable with how I sounded. I hated what the strokes had done to my voice. But then I told myself that lending my voice to a public service announcement on stroke was far different than anchoring a mainstream newscast, and that my voice was strong enough to pass in this setting.

Meanwhile, Denise came to the conclusion early on that I should get out and circulate among my peers, to help reestablish my confidence and provide an incentive for me to work even harder in therapy. This was probably a good idea, although here again I didn't think I was ready. I didn't want my local news colleagues to see me like this. Not now. Not yet. I wasn't ready for them to see me at my most vulnerable. I thought once again of Dick Clark on that New Year's Eve broadcast and reminded myself that television is a tough business. In newsrooms across the country, people are always sizing you up. We climb on talent and the missteps of others. And to complicate things, I was the network news guy. I'd just come to town the year before, with all kinds of fanfare. It was hard enough to join a local newsroom after the kind of career I'd enjoyed at CBS. It's a difficult adjustment, to go from a seasoned veteran to a guy who could hardly talk. I spoke s-o-o-o-o-o slowly, people were biting their lips to keep from finishing my sentences for me. It used to be that I could talk rings around everyone else in the room. Now all I could do was try their patience—and their friendship.

But, of course, I underestimated my colleagues and myself. People couldn't have been more understanding, once I gave them the chance, and I couldn't have been more moved by the warm welcome I received each time I put myself out there. I have Denise to thank for the initial push to go back to the station. She knew how tentative I was about returning to the newsroom, but she convinced me that a visit was just what I needed. She said people got the wrong impression when they talked to me on the phone because I sounded worse than I was. When they saw me in person, they knew I was doing okay. Physically, I was actually doing great. I had lost about twenty-five pounds. People told me I looked ten years younger. Once I started to move around, you could definitely tell that I was moving a little more slowly, a little more tentatively, but Denise was kind enough not to point this out to me.

She hatched a plan. She set it up so I would go back to work—not to resume my job just yet, but to go down to the station to let everyone see how I was doing. She ran it by my news director, Skip Valet, and my general manager, Henry Maldonado, and they thought it was a fine idea. Me, I was a little worried about it, but I went along because I thought it would help me in my fight back.

I had no idea it would be a party. I thought I'd quietly slip in between newscasts, shake a couple hands, and then leave. But there was a giant banner draped across the newsroom that said, "Welcome back, Mark." A cameraman who'd been at WKMG for fourteen years told me he'd never seen a party at the station quite like the one they threw for me. Skip put a microphone on me before I stepped inside. I thought, Why do I need a mike? But I didn't say anything. Then we walked in to thunderous applause. I couldn't believe my eyes and ears. People were lined up just to give me a hug. It seemed like everyone who worked at the station was there to greet me. There was cake and other goodies. There was a pile of mail bundled by my desk—get-well-soon wishes, from viewers and former colleagues.

After a while, Skip quieted the room and gave a nice speech. Then Denise took the mike and gave a nice speech. I think Henry spoke as well. Then they threw to me, and I struggled through a few words. I wouldn't exactly call what I said a nice speech—I can't even recall what I said!—but everybody was quiet as I spoke. Nobody tried to rush me, or to finish my sentences for me. There was warmth and good feeling all around, and a couple tears as well. I was overcome. I looked around the room at all these smiling, welcoming faces. I saw my coanchor, Jacquie Sosa. I saw my morning weatherman, Larry Mowry. It was the first time I'd seen them since my strokes.

It felt great to be back—but I wasn't *all the way back*, and it took a day like this to keep me pressing ahead.

My rehabilitation didn't end once my sessions at BIRC ran their course. I continued with my speech, occupational, and physical therapy for several months, and along the way I added some new therapies if I thought they might help. In May, about six months after my strokes, I began a five-day-a-week course of oxygen treatments that lasted for several weeks. I heard about it at a dinner party at Henry Maldonado's house, from a woman who had suffered a stroke ten years earlier and found the treatments helpful. She told me that the convention in the rest of the developed world is to put stroke patients on oxygen right away, but that here in the United States doctors tended to disregard its benefits.

I thought, What do I have to lose?

It occurred to me that we've become conditioned to expect our cure-alls in pill form. No one wants to do the hard work to get better. No one wants to be the first person to try a new or unconventional treatment. We'd rather take the easy way around. That's why there's a new diet every day, when we all know the key to losing weight is to eat less and exercise more. People believe it's easier to lower their blood pressure and cholesterol levels through pills than through diet. But sometimes you have to look outside yourself and beyond established medical practice if you mean to get past whatever it is that's ailing you.

Sometimes, the medical establishment won't pay for such an aggressive approach. The oxygen treatments were expensive—about $160 a pop—but I was determined to follow through on it, and fortunate enough to be able to pay for them myself. The treatments consisted of me getting into a hyperbaric chamber for an hour each day. I could only wear cotton clothes inside the chamber. At first, I stayed awake during these sessions, but after a while I got so comfortable in there I would fall asleep. I could close my eyes and drift off. There was a television, so when I couldn't sleep I watched *SportsCenter* on ESPN.

Most of the patients in the Orlando clinic where I received the oxygen treatments were children, so I met a lot of moms in the waiting room. They asked a lot of questions, because they all had parents or grandparents or friends recovering from stroke, and most of them had never heard about the related benefits of oxygen. But the benefits were immediately apparent. The pure oxygen went straight to the brain. I found that I left the chamber each day walking a little more confidently. I was a little stronger on my feet. My stamina was greater. Also, I felt like I was thinking more clearly. And according to Denise at least, my speech was quicker, and cleaner.

At this late stage in my rehab and recovery, I looked to Denise for cues as to how I was doing. There was only so much I could see for myself in the mirror, or in the eyes of others. She was honest with me in this regard, which was both a good thing and a bad thing. It was good because I could count on her for an accurate assessment. It was bad because I didn't always want to hear what she had to say. For example, about eighteen months into my recovery, someone asked Denise if she thought I was all the way back, if I was as fully present in her life and in our relationship as I had been before my strokes. She answered quite candidly that I wasn't. Not yet.

Denise didn't say what she said to be mean. She was just being honest, and it took hearing it back for me to realize there were some new hurdles for me to clear, some I hadn't even thought about. That "guy" Denise was talking about was still here. I was still me. It's just that it took a little effort for me to bring him into the room. If a joke alighted in my head, or a quick response, it was sometimes too much of an effort to put it out there. My mind was once again as sharp as it had ever been, but I couldn't download my thoughts and musings as effortlessly as I had once been able to— so these jabs and retorts just withered on the vine. It was something to work on, I told myself. Always, there was something to work on.

My speech was a worry. I had always been able to "hear" my voice inside my head, but I couldn't do so after my strokes. I didn't recognize it, so I had to rely on the feedback I took in from people I could trust. It was always nice to hear such positive feedback, but only if I knew it was offered honestly, objectively. With my voice, I could always speak into a tape recorder and play it back to hear how I sounded. I did this for a while, until I heard myself on the air being interviewed and I began to like how my voice sounded. The pitch was getting back to where it used to be, so I started working on the fluidity of my speech.

I also tried acupuncture. For some reason, my insurance

company covered these treatments, but not my oxygen treatments. All I had to pay was my $15 co-pay, so I started going twice a week in June 2006, about seven months into my recovery. Before I went, my right hand was swollen. Acupuncture helped to reduce the swelling. Before I went, my voice was still high-pitched. Acupuncture helped to lower it. I had needles under my throat, on the top of my head, in my right forearm, and in my right leg. I must have looked a sight, but I didn't care. If someone told me a certain kind of treatment or therapy might work, I gave it a shot, and now I recommend acupuncture to anyone who's had a stroke. In some cases it works, and in some it doesn't, but we have to keep open to the possibility that Far Eastern medicine can help Western patients. The treatment doesn't discriminate. It doesn't care where you're from or what you've been conditioned to believe.

I even tried laser treatments to reduce the swelling in my right hand and fingers. My insurance covered this, too, and I think it worked. I can't say for certain, because I began the treatments while I was taking acupuncture, so it could have been one or the other or both working in combination. Anyway, the swelling went down. I didn't have time to focus on treatments sequentially and wait for each one to work. I was too busy trying everything, and pushing myself, and working overtime to regain what stroke had taken from me.

I continued with my physical therapy until August, almost ten months in, and I kept up with my speech and occupational therapy regimens for some months after that. I was relentless in my approach—and here again, my approach is not for everybody. It worked for me, but it was really, really hard.

Early on, I talked about returning to work in the spring, at least on a limited schedule, but then spring rolled around and my voice was still far from broadcast-worthy, so I set a new goal for myself. I would be back in the summer. After that, it was the fall. I reminded myself that I wasn't ready. As I wrote earlier, the folks at WKMG couldn't have been nicer about it, or more understanding. At first, they were holding my job for me, thinking it would only be a matter of months before I was back in the anchor seat, but when that didn't happen they had to fill the spot. I understood that. They had a station to run and a news team to promote. They couldn't hold my seat indefinitely. I couldn't blame them. All I could do was keep reading to myself, aloud, for an hour each day, strengthening my voice. I'd read from a newspaper or a magazine. Sometimes I'd read from the laptop because it could imitate a teleprompter. And I made it a special point to read to Miles and Griffin every night. That became our thing. It was a great way for us to spend time together at the end of each day, with the side benefit that I was working on my voice.

Soon I was back on television as spokesperson for "Good Neighbor 6," a series of spots highlighting good health. I covered general health issues, as well as stroke-specific stories, and even got to talk on the air. It was the first time I'd been on television in a working capacity since the strokes. I'd been interviewed on television. I'd been a guest. But here I was, back doing my thing—holding my own microphone, so to speak. Denise also got involved as the front person for a documentary-type special called *Miracle of Love*, which showed my ordeal through her eyes. The special, which was seen locally in Orlando, in prime time, ended up winning its time slot and its night.

The hard work of rehab and recovery was made easier by the new friends I was making in the stroke community. It's funny, because I never really knew anyone who'd had a stroke, and now here I was running into stroke patients and stroke experts left and right. Denise and I had a similar experience when the boys were born. Parents with twins kept popping up like mushrooms after a rainstorm. Now it was the same thing all over again. People who are touched by stroke are everywhere, I was learning. All it takes is going through it to open yourself up to it. There are even two national umbrella organizations for stroke. There's the American Stroke Association and the National Stroke Association. It's not like the American Cancer Society, where there's only one organization to advance the cause. We've got two, and I count this as a giant positive. Isn't it better to have two boards, two sources of information for patients and families, two fund-raising arms, two awareness campaigns? You can reach a lot more people and make a bigger impact, which is why I happily agreed to work for each group. My thinking was, they're both doing good things, they're both out in front on issues relating to stroke, so I might as well lend my voice to each organization.

One of the big steps in my recovery was my return appearance on *The Early Show* on CBS. I'd been talking to my old friends at the network since I was in the hospital, and people like Cathy Black, my old entertainment producer and close friend, and Harry Smith, my longtime buddy, kept telling me to come by the set whenever I felt strong enough to do so. I held out the prospect like a carrot on a stick. I looked forward to the day like you couldn't imagine. I finally took them up on their offer in September, 2006, nine months after I left the hospital. Here again, I hadn't expected any kind of grand welcome, but CBS was always good about taking care of one of its own. They brought me onto the set for a reunion with Harry after showing a taped piece on me that focused on my comeback from stroke. I'd known beforehand that this was the plan, but it still caught me unprepared. How do you prepare for something like this? It's like being on an episode of *This Is Your Life*. There were hugs and well-wishing all around. Everyone stopped what they were doing to give me a warm, meaningful hello: Julie Chen, Hannah Storm, René Syler, and Dave Price; the stagehands, the camera guys, and the producers; the director, whom I knew when he was just starting out. Harry looked on and said, "Talk about lighting up a room!"

I even got a congratulatory phone call after the segment aired from the senior President Bush. He happened to catch the show and wanted to touch base, and to tell me how well he thought I was doing.

I was thrilled, and not just about the presidential phone call. Mostly I was thrilled to be back on my old set, surrounded by my old colleagues, even though I was not quite ready to return to the airwaves in any kind of full-time role. Mostly, I was overjoyed to send such a positive, hopeful message to the national stroke community that there is indeed life after stroke, and that even in the most extreme cases patients can expect to recover pieces of their old lives and graft them onto whatever new experiences lie in wait.

Indeed, this was my plan going forward.

LIFE BEFORE STROKE: *Orlando*

As I wrote earlier, it took a long time for me and Denise to finally get together. Right now, we're deep into happily-ever-after mode, although for a while it seemed my stroke might have something to say about the *happily* part (not to mention the *ever-after* part), and for a while before that it seemed we might never wind up with each other at all.

The long-story-short version of my marriage to Linda Boston is that it didn't last. We parted on good terms, and I started to spend more and more time on the road for CBS. I liked being married, but now I found that I liked being single. I checked in with Denise when my marriage ended, but she was involved with someone else. I told myself this was for the best. Things were so busy on the morning show, and my hours so crazy, that I didn't think I had time for another relationship—but somehow another relationship came calling. Literally. Her name was Judith Lonsdale. We met over the phone. I worked with her sister, and she decided to fix us up, only Judy lived in Los Angeles.

She sent me a picture. She knew what I looked like from television. I knew what she looked like from a snapshot of her wearing bug-eyed sunglasses so big you couldn't see her face. She thought it was funny, sending me a picture like that. It was.

We got married soon after. Judy moved to New York, but I was still on the road a good deal. The job was the job. It wasn't about to change. I bounced from city to city, interviewing celebrities, broadcasting from state fairs, performing outrageous stunts, reporting the weather. I had become the face of CBS in the morning. The producers played into that. They looked to feature me in certain feel-good, signature broadcasts. For example, for my fortieth birthday, they hosted an on-air surprise party. They taped a number of prominent people wishing me a happy birthday. Mary Hart from *Entertainment Tonight*. Willie Nelson. Aretha Franklin sang a song for me. It was a real celebration. The highlight was the taped appearance of my boyhood idol, Bob Gibson. The producers had asked Judy who they should ask to participate, and Bob's was the one name she gave. She knew that in 1964, when I was living in Berlin, I pitched for a Little League team called the Cardinals, the same year Bob Gibson was mowing down the Yankees in the World Series for the real Cardinals.

I almost fell on the floor when I saw Bob. It was a giant thrill. I had already met presidents and Oscar winners and bestselling authors, but nothing could touch this. When Bob published his autobiography, I pleaded with my boss to let me travel to his home in Omaha to interview him. We became friends. I played at his charity golf tournaments. We went to dinner. He and his wife, Wendy, came to see us in Orlando more than once after my stroke.

At some point, Judy and I decided to start a family, but we had some trouble in this area. We jumped through all kinds of hoops. Then one day I heard about an organization in Florida that provides neonatal care to mothers who decide early on to give their child up for adoption. At the time, I was friendly with Tom Cruise. He had adopted his first two children through the state of Florida, and he was the first one to tell me how the laws in Florida were particularly friendly to adoptive parents.

We flew down to Florida during hurricane season, but it would take a lot more than a hurricane to keep us from this baby. I took one look at Maya and knew right away she was my daughter. She was only ten days old.

Unfortunately, Maya was one of the last things Judy and I got right. We separated about three years later. It killed me to do that to Maya, especially because she was still too young to understand.

Meanwhile, Denise and I were on-again and off-again and back-and-forth and all over the place. One of us was always married or otherwise engaged. Just as it had when we first met when Denise was still in high school, our timing sucked. And then, suddenly, it didn't. I called her as soon as my divorce was final. She was living in Orlando. I got her answering machine. I stole a line from *Risky Business.* I said, "This is my what-the-fuck phone call." I said, "This is not about being boyfriend and girlfriend. This is not about me being in New York and you being in Florida. This is about us getting married."

Happily, Denise agreed to see me. The deal was I would come to Orlando and we would talk. She was still involved with someone, so that was all that could happen. We were both clear on this, but I figured this was a start. I took a hotel room at the airport. She came by, and we talked. We played backgammon. We drank Jack and Gingers. We cried, and wondered what was wrong with us that we could never get it together to get together. In the morning, I flew back to New York and went to Tiffany's to shop for an engagement ring. Denise went home to her boyfriend and broke it off. The next weekend I flew back down to Florida and asked her to marry me. I actually dropped to one knee and proposed, just like in the movies.

A couple months later we were married and living in New York and talking about babies. She had a daughter, Jenna, from a previous marriage, and I had Maya, but we wanted to have a child together. Thanks to in vitro, we were soon trying, but not before the bottom fell out on my network news career. After fifteen years at CBS, the network decided not to renew my contract. This was a shock, because I had survived every other shake-up the morning show had seen during my tenure. I'd stepped down as coanchor to make way for Bryant Gumbel, who was meant to be the savior for CBS in the morning, but now after only two years Bryant was out. Jane Clayson was out as cohost. For a while, it looked like I might stay on to once again provide a kind of continuity for viewers during the reshuffling of talent, but then all of a sudden it didn't.

This, too, was the life of a network morning show personality.

I was forty-nine years old, newly married, and out of a job. We weren't worried about money, but I needed to work, so I started going out on interviews. I went to MSNBC, in Secaucus, New Jersey. I went to WMAQ-TV in Chicago. I went to Los Angeles to interview for a spot on the syndicated entertainment show *Extra*. I told the executive producer I didn't care who an actor or actress was sleeping with. I just cared what was in their mind and in their heart. The executive producer said, "Well, we care who they're sleeping with." I didn't get the job.

It was during this job-hunting period that the in vitro took. Denise called one day with the good news that she was pregnant with twins. Our boys, Miles and Griffin, were born in September 2003. (We gave Miles the middle name Gibson, in honor of my friend Bob.) All of a sudden, a job didn't seem so important. My focus changed. I started going out on interviews at local television stations, in markets like Raleigh, North Carolina, thinking it would be a good place to raise our growing family.

When the job came up at WKMG, the CBS affiliate in Orlando, I was very happy. Denise had uprooted herself from Orlando to join me in New York, so it seemed fitting that we double back onto her turf. I met Skip Valet and Henry Maldonado for dinner and came away thinking, These people are very nice. In fact, everything about the job and the city seemed very nice.

I thought, We can make a life here. A fresh start.

CONSTRAINT

It's Getting Better All the Time

Everybody has a story. It doesn't have to be about stroke. It can be about anything. It can be about a small thing like breaking a leg and coming back, or a big thing like surviving cancer or a heart attack. Whatever you're suffering, whatever you and your family are going through, if you put it out there for the rest of the world you'll hear back how the rest of the world handled it.

I'm sharing my story here because I want stroke survivors to know that they're not alone. That stroke can affect anyone. That stroke doesn't discriminate. We'd all do well to keep open to the experiences of those around us, especially when it comes to stroke. There is no one path to a full recovery, just as there is no shortcut. I knew this in theory, going into my ordeal, but it took reaching through to the other side to know it full well. Indeed, there are so many different therapies out there, so many different agencies devoted to stroke patients and their families, so many different theories and caregivers and plans of attack that Denise and I have often wondered how to make sense of it all. What we've realized, finally, is that you can't. You'll go crazy trying to keep up with every diet or exercise regimen designed to reduce the risk of stroke or to speed recovery. You'll fill your days consulting with every doctor and therapist who claims to have discovered some new and improved method, and your nights worrying that there might be something more you could do. All you can do is keep your eyes open for a treatment plan that makes sense for you and fits into your lifestyle.

It was with this mind-set that I ran into an old high school friend named Ken Peck. He was putting on a charity golf tournament, and he reached out to me to help spread the word. We got to talking. Ken had lost both his legs to a rare blood disease and now worked for a prosthetic company. He'd heard his fair share of stories, of course, and he told me one about a guy who'd had a stroke about four years earlier. The guy was a big golfer, and he'd recovered a good deal of mobility, but he'd reached the stage where his doctors and therapists were telling him he'd gone about as far as he could go. For the longest time, that was the conventional wisdom when it came to stroke. The golfer was told that whatever he could do at that point, he would continue to do; whatever he could not, he would most likely never be able to do again. Unfortunately, he couldn't hit a golf ball. This was a problem, because the only thing this guy wanted to do was hit golf balls. He lived for his time on the course. He could drive and shave and do almost everything else, but he was pretty depressed about not playing golf. To him, nothing was as important.

Finally, the frustrated golfer heard about a progressive form of therapy known as constraint therapy, or mitt therapy. It was based on a simple concept: you constrain your stronger hand in such a way that you force your weaker hand to overcome its weakness. In theory, it's a lot like a baseball coach who teaches his players to bat from the opposite side of the plate, because he knows switch-hitters have a better shot at reaching the majors. You strengthen your "off" hand by relying exclusively on it. Naturally, the frustrated golfer signed on for this therapy, and within a couple weeks he was back to playing golf.

I'd heard about this type of therapy when I was at Lucerne, and later on when I was rehabbing at BIRC, but it wasn't offered at either of those places, and there were so many other treatment options that I guess I let it slide. There weren't enough hours in the day to pursue every course of treatment. Plus, I was making good progress with my various therapists. That's how it went with me. When something worked, I was inclined to keep at it, even if there were some pieces missing in my recovery. You catch yourself thinking there'll always be time to work on the other stuff later.

Now, though, it was the spring of 2007, and I was almost a year and a half removed from my stroke. The time had come to work on some of that "other stuff." Like that frustrated golfer, I worried I might have reached some kind of plateau. I didn't have a golf game to worry about. My worry was my voice, and I continued to make gains in this area, sounding more and more like my old self each day, speaking with greater ease and fluidity and less slurring. I had more energy. But it was the rest of the package that now had me worried. My biggest concern was that I didn't have the strength or dexterity in my right hand that I felt I needed to get my life back to where it was.

I caught myself starting to think that the mobility I once took for granted in my right hand, my *dominant* hand, would never completely return. Every task I willed my right hand to perform was a struggle. Some I could manage; some I could not. Most I just reassigned to my left hand, which was easier than powering through and forcing my right hand to do the work. As a result, in the year and a half since my stroke, my left hand had gotten much stronger. I'd learned to compensate. I taught myself to write with my left hand, to dial a phone with my left hand, to brush my teeth with my left hand.

Because of Ken, I started making some calls, which eventually took me to a facility called Village Rehabilitation

Specialists in Lady Lake, Florida, outside Orlando, and a physical therapist who worked there named Camille Magnuson. She came highly recommended. Her patients loved her. And every last one of them reported that they were doing better since they worked with Camille—far better than they had come to believe was possible. Together, we discussed whether constraint therapy might work for me. Almost immediately, we determined that it would.

On a personal level, I was sold right away. All it took was meeting with Camille and learning about her painstaking and thoroughgoing approach to know that this could be just the push I needed to get me beyond my plateau. It was based on such a simple theory, I thought, how could it not work? I looked over the Village literature and noticed that one of the exercises they recommended for certain patients was crawling. That's right, crawling. The idea is that by dropping down on all fours and advancing with the right hand and left knee, and then the left hand and right knee, you strengthen your upper body and your scapular stability. (That's your shoulder blade, by the way.) It was not yet clear to me that I was a candidate for this type of exercise, but I was struck by the back-to-basics aspects of it. I mean, what could be more basic than crawling? You have to crawl before you walk, and walk before you run, so I thought any rehab outfit that advocates such a fundamental approach was okay by me.

One of the first things we had to do was carve out some time in my now busy schedule, because the therapy required six-hour sessions for fourteen consecutive days. (It was also an hour drive—one way.) It was a big commitment, in virtually every respect. Happily, my health insurance company agreed to pay for it, because it was a big financial commitment as well. The approval wasn't a slam dunk, though. Denise went back and forth with Aetna for months on this, because they were willing to pay for the constraint therapy, but they wanted me to do it at a rehab facility closer to Orlando. I was determined to work with Camille at Village. The total bill came to about eight thousand dollars, so it was a lot of money, and Aetna kept turning me down. They said the program at the facility closer to my home was just as good and a lot less expensive. I couldn't really argue with them, but I had heard great things about Village, and I was really sold on Camille, so we kept pressing for the approval.

For months and months, we kept pressing. At some point, I got so tired of waiting for Aetna to agree to the therapy I decided to just pay for it myself. The constraint therapy was something I felt I really needed, as well as something I felt I could afford. So I found a three-week hole in my calendar, to account for the weekends. This, too, was no easy task, because it wasn't just my calendar I had to worry about. It was Denise's, and Maya's, and Jenna's, and the boys'. I'd be out of pocket for virtually every piece of weekday family business.

We set it up for the middle of June. The program started with an extensive orientation, and a day or two before I was due to go in for it we learned that Aetna would pay for the therapy after all. I thought, Well, it's about time. I also thought, Okay, I'm not the only one who thinks this is a good idea. It was a great relief when the insurance person checked in with my approval—not only because I was worried about the cost, but also because I wanted to be sure I was doing the right thing. Sometimes, with health insurance, it's not just the money that matters to patients. It's the validation. It's knowing that the course of treatment you've selected and the health-care provider you've chosen have been endorsed by the people who consider these things for a living. I was going for it anyway, but it was nice to be able to go for it with the corroboration of a second opinion.

The Village orientation consisted of a series of strength measures in my right hand and my left hand. Camille had me squeeze a contraption that measured the poundage I could handle on each side. I was supposed to squeeze it as hard as I could, and then to hold it for as long as I could. I imagined what my measurements would have been before the stroke, when I was fit and strong. My left hand checked in at about ninety pounds. My right hand was about seventy-five. Camille said that if the therapy went well, she could help me build my right hand to over one hundred pounds. It didn't sound like a big number, or a big jump, but she assured me it would make all the difference. She also tested the strength in my fingers. She did this by having me squeeze a small weight between two fingers. Thumb to forefinger. Thumb to ring finger. Forefinger to middle finger. She had me do every possible combination, and then we moved to groups of three fingers. At first, she left the pinky out of it. She told me to worry about the rest of my hand first, and that the pinky wasn't so much about strength as positioning.

The idea with all these measurements was to establish a baseline for my abilities before beginning the therapy, but already with this opening round of weight and strength assessment exercises I could see there would be some benefit. I was working muscles and combinations of muscles that had been dormant for over a year, and I could feel that there was a lot of hard work ahead—work I perhaps should have been doing for months by this point. I had been so focused on my voice, and on the basics in terms of physical therapy, that I really hadn't been thinking aggressively about the rest of my body.

The actual therapy began on a Monday. My sessions started on the wrist exercycle. It was similar to the machine I used back at BIRC, and designed to work the upper body. At first, I did fifteen minutes in each direction—and it was exhausting! I didn't think there'd be anything to it, but I couldn't have managed another minute. Each day, Camille would have me do a little more on the exercycle, to where by the end of the first week I was doing almost an hour. It was meant to be a warm-up, but at the other end I was ready for a nap.

In truth, I didn't mind the fatigue or the exhaustion so much as the boredom. Even when I went to the gym before my stroke, I was never an exercise bicycle kind of guy. Like most people, I need to be distracted when I work out, and here at Village I found my distraction out the window. I passed the time counting cars as they drove past the clinic. I made a game of it in my head. I counted cars versus trucks and vans. For some reason, I determined twenty was the magic number. In baseball, twenty wins is the mark of a great season for a starting pitcher, so I told myself I'd have to get to twenty cars before I got to twenty trucks and vans. I kept score. I would go 20–15, or 20–7, or 20–19. At certain times of day, the trucks and vans would win out. At other times, later in the morning it would be the cars in a romp. I don't think I ever "pitched a shutout"—that is, counting twenty cars before a single truck or van came down the street—but I came close.

Music was another great distraction. They usually kept the radio dialed to a classic rock station, and I'd lose myself in all these wonderful songs I used to play when I was working in Baltimore, Detroit, and Chicago. The Romantics, Journey, Styx—this was the music I built my career upon. I loved these songs. The classic rock from the '60s and '70s was something else. The Beatles, the Stones, Led Zeppelin—those were the artists I grew up on as a kid, but for some reason the station they listened to at Village played a lot of '80s music. Boston, Bob Seger, Foreigner. . . .

Camille was busy adding those few grueling minutes on the exercycle to my pregame warm-up each morning, and each time I felt like quitting a great song would come on and I'd kick things up a notch. I was a country music fan, thanks to my mother, and a friend of Garth Brooks. He was one of those artists who wouldn't be pigeonholed by labels or genres. One of his songs came on one morning, and I smiled to myself. I thought, Any day that starts with Garth Brooks is bound to be a good day.

The song was "The Dance," and it took me back because I'd interviewed Garth a bunch of times when I was at CBS. We got along great. The first time was when he was just starting out. A lot of times, these artists are out on the road, promoting a new album, and they're being interviewed by people who couldn't sing a single one of their songs. But Garth enjoyed the fact that I enjoyed his music. We developed a fine friendship, which meant a great deal to me. When he was named "Artist of the Decade" for the 1990s, he gave me a special ring. He had these beautiful rings made up to give to his band members, his record company pals, and other members of his professional family, almost like the way a baseball team distributes World Series rings to the entire organization after winning a championship. He only gave three rings to people outside his circle: Jay Leno, Nancy O'Dell (from *Access Hollywood*), and me. It was his way of thanking us. I was really touched by the gesture—and the ring quickly became one of my most treasured possessions.

Whenever I wear that ring, it reminds me of the time Garth bailed me out of a tough spot. All the morning shows were in Orlando to cover the twentieth anniversary of Walt Disney World. It was a huge celebration. We had a segment booked with Patti LaBelle that was to be a highlight of that morning's broadcast, but unfortunately Patti got sick at the last minute and had to pull out. That kind of thing happened all the time in morning television. As the CBS News entertainment reporter, it fell to me to hustle up a replacement, so I found the Disney promotions guy and asked him who else was in town for the celebration. The first person he mentioned was Garth Brooks.

I said, "Stop right there."

The guy said, "Well, maybe you should hear a couple more names. I don't think Garth is doing any interviews." Already, my friend Garth had turned down *Today*, *Good Morning America*, and *Live with Regis and Kathie Lee*.

I said, "Just tell him it's for Mark McEwen."

The promo guy shrugged his shoulders like he thought I was sending him on a fool's errand, but then he returned a short time later with a look of genuine astonishment. He said, "Let me tell you how this went. I talked to Garth's people. I said, 'I know you've turned everybody down, but Mark McEwen...' They interrupted me before I could finish. They said, 'Mark? We'll do it.'"

Sure enough, Garth showed up on our set to do the interview, and he couldn't have been nicer about it. He's always been there for me. He called the house as soon as he heard about my stroke. He was really calming. He has this way about him that really helps you focus on what's important. He gets right to the heart of the matter. He told me to get the best rehab therapists I could find. I told him I was doing just that. It's always a great pick-me-up when I hear his voice on the other end of the phone, just as it was a great pick-me-up to hear his song on the radio that morning early on during my stint at Village. It wasn't like me to read too much into such a small coincidence as hearing a friend's song on the radio, but it was an uplifting thing, to listen to my friend Garth as I went through my workout.

There was another personal connection that found me at Village, and this one freaked me out a little—in a good way, I suppose. I met a woman there named Dolores. She was another patient. She was older than me. When we were introduced to each other, she told me her name, and I asked her how she spelled it because that was my mother's name. Growing up, whenever my mother ran across another Dolores, she always asked her how she spelled her name, and I thought it was funny that I did, too. I did it without even thinking about it.

The woman replied that she spelled her name with an *o*. I said, "That's how my mother spelled it."

We chatted for a while to break the monotony of our exercise routines, and this Dolores let on that she had lived in Berlin when John F. Kennedy came to visit. I said, "So did I."

Then I thought, That's odd. There was nothing else about this woman that reminded me of my mother, but the spelling of her name and this unlikely Berlin connection were enough to leave me thinking she was some kind of angel, sent to watch over me as I worked myself back to whole. I felt the same way when Garth Brooks came in over the radio.

Of course, the real work of physical therapy had nothing to do with angels or coincidences. It had to do with sweat and discipline and focus. It had to do with setting goals and rising to meet them. And it had to do with believing that there was still something you could do to set things right. Almost all of the work I did at Village was concentrated on my upper body. Even before I started my constraint therapy sessions, I was walking a little more like my old self each day, but with my balance still leaving a little something to be desired. It would be some time before I could move with the same spring in my step I had always enjoyed. Nevertheless, Camille said we wouldn't focus on my legs, because I was on them all the time. They would get a good workout anyway, she said, and so the right hand was my main focus—and since my right hand was connected to my right shoulder, that's where we started.

Camille put my left hand in a mitt, so I wouldn't even think about using it to complete any of the tasks she laid out for me. This was the *constraint* part of the therapy. Apparently, if I merely willed myself to use only my right hand, my brain would still send out signals to my left hand to help accomplish each task, and my body would be inclined to cheat or short-circuit the therapy, but if my left hand was encased in a big mitt it would be completely unavailable to me and my brain would begin to recognize that. It was like an oven mitt, with no thumb. When it was wrapped in the mitt, I could not have used that hand to unscrew a lightbulb or pick up a newspaper or turn a doorknob, so I had no choice but to put my right hand to work.

The mitt was a bit confusing for my twins, Miles and Griffin. Part of the therapy was I had to wear it at home, and when I did the boys didn't know what to make of it. Miles, for one, took one look at his old man and pointed at my gloved hand and said, "Boo-boo."

I said, "No, Miles. No boo-boo."

"Boo-boo," he said again.

"No, Miles," I tried, "it's not a boo-boo. It's just something daddy has to wear to get stronger."

Miles was very interested in this, because this was a boo-boo he could see. The boo-boo in my head was a little harder for him to grasp. Remember, he was only three years old at the time, so his reactions made sense. To him, this was just a big bandage, a hurt he could kiss and make all better, so after a while I stopped correcting him. If he wanted it to be a boo-boo, it would be a boo-boo.

The work was hard. Walter and my other physical therapists had put me through some heavy-duty exercises at Lucerne and BIRC, but that was mostly to get me up and moving again. This was different. With Camille, I had to factor in a certain level of frustration and learn how to deal with that frustration, because a lot of what she had me doing was simple, dexterity-type stuff. She worked on strengthening my shoulders, but also on strengthening my fingers. The way to do this, she said, was to repeat certain fine motor tasks. For example, I had to place a series of objects on a Velcro strip that Camille held high, and once the objects were in place I had to take them off one by one. She had me do this over and over.

There was another exercise with clothespins that was especially difficult. It was maddening, actually—at least at first. I had to take a series of colored clothespins from a box and place them on a wire Camille strung out before me. Some of the clothespins were more difficult to open than others, and the color correlated to the tension or resistance. The hardest ones were the black ones. I sorted them on Camille's order, according to whatever sequence she set out for me. This, too, I did over and over, with the sequence changing each time.

I also worked with a board with a series of large screws, and I had to twist them in and out of the grooves—over and over.

In case you missed it, *over and over* was one of the big themes of this place. It wasn't enough to do a thing once or twice; we did it into the ground, and then we did it a couple times more. It was the repetition, Camille said, that helped to train my muscle memory for each task and to rewire my brain to help return my right hand to its dominant status—although, frankly, some of these tasks had almost nothing to do with any real-life chore I'd ever be called on to complete. I'll give an example: I didn't think I'd ever need to move grains of rice from a bowl to a plastic cup—but that's just what Camille had me doing. Over and over, of course. The kicker here was that I had to use a pair of tweezers to lift the grains and transfer them. It was busywork, just, but Camille assured me it was busywork with a purpose.

The cups were arranged in rows, and I had to fill them to the brim without spilling a single grain of rice. If it sounds easy, it's not. (Go ahead and try it with your strongest hand, and see how easy it is!) It was probably the most pointless, most frustrating task any of my therapists laid out for me over the course of my rehabilitation, but at the same time there was something about it that appealed to me. I caught myself thinking it was very Zen, very soothing in its pointlessness, and as I worked at it I lapsed into a kind of Zen zone. Nothing was more important than this pointless task at hand. And nothing would keep me from filling these rows of cups with grains of rice. In fact, the first time I finished filling the cups, I felt such an enormous rush of accomplishment, and then right away I felt almost silly for feeling so proud, given what it was I had actually accomplished, because of course this was something an extremely patient child could have accomplished, and because when I was finished the rice would just get dumped back into the bowl.

For a real-life chore that gave me some trouble at first, there was Maya's old iPod. She got a new one for Christmas that year, and decided I was ready to greet the digital age and put her old one to use. I couldn't argue. What dad wants to tell his eleven-year-old daughter that he'd rather listen to the radio or to old-fashioned CDs than to an iPod? The only problem was I had some trouble getting my right hand to work the iPod's unusual push-wheel touch pad. For a couple months, I left it sitting on my desk, and whenever Maya asked about it I came up with some excuse why I wasn't using it. Now, with my left hand entombed in my mitt, my right hand could only fumble across the iPod controls, and I counted myself lucky to get the thing to work at all. But I made it a challenge. I worked at it. Maya helped me figure out how to download some of my own songs, and that gave me some incentive. If you've spent any time at all with an iPod, you'll know exactly why I was having trouble with the push-wheel controls, but I stayed with it and eventually mastered the machine to where I started using it during rehab each day.

I did another series of exercises with weights on my arm, to make the tasks more difficult and to build muscle mass at the same time. Sometimes the exercise was all about strength conditioning, like one where I had to carry a bucket laden with five-pound weights from one side of the building to another. Man, that was hard! I got home that night and I couldn't lift my arms over my head to get out of my T-shirt.

It took being in all these different kinds of therapies, doing all these different kinds of exercises to realize that therapists want you to succeed. Absolutely, they do. This is a generalization, I know, but it's not a line of work for people who think negatively. (And for patients who think negatively, it doesn't promise a whole lot of success, I don't care what kind of therapy you're talking about.) I look back now on the dozens of different therapists who worked with me at various points in my rehabilitations, and this was one thing every one of them had in common. They liked their jobs, and they liked it when their patients persevered and saw improvement. It made their day.

In success, it made mine too, and at the end of each day I tried to measure my own progress in my head, to weigh where I was against where I had been. Typically, I couldn't see any change, because that's how it is when you're living through any kind of transformation. The change is gradual. It's like watching hair grow. But guess what? Eventually it grows. Eventually, you get a little stronger, and after that you get a little stronger still.

The mitt was key, because it prohibited me from using my left hand. The deal was I was supposed to wear it throughout the rest of the day, after I left Village, and all through the evening. I'd take it off to drive, but other than that I kept it on, and it forced me to use keys with my right hand, to open doors with my right hand, to hold a cup of coffee, brush my teeth, and so on. Camille told me that as long as it had taken for me to relearn how to do all these things with my left hand after my stroke, that's how long it would take for my brain to remember to use my right hand going forward.

Whatever Camille threw at me, I tried to handle with grace and good cheer. I don't think I complained once, the whole time I was in her care. I don't even think I allowed myself to really feel frustrated. There were small frustrations, but they were manageable frustrations. There was nothing I couldn't get past. One thing you need to know about me is that I'm hard on myself. No one is harder on me than me. I think you have to be, to get through something like this. So I would just go forward, no matter what. I was like Frodo in *The Lord of the Rings*, who said, "I will take the ring even though I don't know the way."

Know the way? I couldn't tell you up from down or east from west. But I knew I wanted to get better. And I was.

HOME

And Who Knows Which Is Which and Who Is Who

I t's been nearly two years since my strokes, and I'm feeling great. I continue to make progress, although lately progress has been slow. The days of big, transforming improvement are in the past, and yet I continue to improve. I've met a lot of stroke patients who get discouraged by this slowdown in the pace of their recovery, but I take it as a positive. Progress is progress. And you don't need to be a traffic reporter to know that slow is better than a standstill.

It used to be that doctors and therapists believed stroke patients could regain their abilities lost to stroke for about six months following their "event," after which they could expect to remain at that level of impairment for the rest of their lives. After that, the benchmark was a year, and then two years. Now, according to the folks I talk to, there is no benchmark. There's no set timeline. You can expect to see gains and improvements at any time, as long as you're prepared to work at it. But you need to be realistic. I can't expect to roll out of bed tomorrow morning and dance the lead in *The Nutcracker*, but with hard work and discipline and sweat and all that good stuff I just might cut it as one of the Sugar Plum Fairies.

The old rules no longer apply—and even if they did, they wouldn't apply to me. I wouldn't let them. You need to be stubborn if you mean to make yourself whole following stroke. It doesn't matter what kind of obstacle you're intent on overcoming, you need to be focused and relentless. You need to be strong. You need to have a plan of attack that maximizes your abilities, with an eye toward achievable results. With stroke, you need to recognize that there is no clock on your recovery, and that true healing takes place along a continuum. It's ongoing. It's evolving. The human body is constantly rejuvenating itself. The rewiring continues well after six months or two years. The relearning continues.

Recovery is a state of mind, I've learned. It's also a constant when it comes to stroke. The pace of recovery might slow after a time, but it definitely continues. On and on and ever forward. As long as you keep putting something into it, you'll keep getting something back out. It's a simple equation. In many ways, it's like the moral to that old fable about the tortoise and the hare—*slow and steady wins the race*—

only here it's not about winning, it's about finishing, so it comes out like this: *slow and steady gets there eventually.*

When you've been knocked to the ground the way I was knocked to the ground, *eventually* looks pretty good.

Whenever I run into someone I haven't seen in months, they congratulate me on my recovery, and I think to myself, I'm not done yet. Hold off on those congratulations, because I'm still just getting there. I've made great gains, to be sure, but there's more work to do. Way more. This is not the finished version of me. This is just Mark McEwen 2.0. There'll be a new, improved version every couple of months.

My watchwords now are: *be healthy.* It terrified me when I first learned that people who suffer strokes are at greater risk of subsequent strokes, but that was before I realized those cautionary numbers typically apply to people who don't change a thing about their diets or lifestyles following the first stroke. Sure, if you live a certain way and eat a certain way that leave you vulnerable to stroke the first time around, you'll be just as vulnerable the second time around if you don't shake things up in your routine. Harry Smith pointed this out to me on the air when he interviewed me on a second visit to the *The Early Show* about eighteen months after my stroke, and I said, "They got me easy the first time. I'm making it harder for them to get me again."

I've changed my diet completely. I eat a lot of fish, salmon especially. I eat a lot of fruits and vegetables. I rarely eat red meat, but I do eat chicken and a lot of turkey. I limit my sugar and salt intake, and I stay away from fried foods. I used to be a fried calamari fiend, but I can't eat it anymore. I mean, I *can*...I just don't. There's a lot of stuff I used to reach for without a thought, but now I'm constantly thinking about what I can eat and what I can't. What I should be eating, and what I should be avoiding. I'll have chocolate from time to time or cake or a fattening kind of meal, because it's okay to indulge every now and then. But I keep my indulgences to a minimum, and that's tough to do with temptation all around. Within a five mile radius of my house, there's a McDonald's, a Burger King, a Taco Bell, and an Arby's. The old me thought nothing about pulling in for a quick bite, or a between-meal snack, but the new me stays away. Now, if I see a drive-thru, I do a drive-by.

Exercise is the foundation for everything else. When I'm at home, I work out at a local gym, about six times a week. For Father's Day, Denise arranged visits for me with a personal trainer at my gym, so I see him twice a week. When I travel, I make sure there's a suitable gym in my hotel before checking in. I do the treadmill, the stationary bike, the free weights. I've got a whole routine. The American Stroke Association recommends at least thirty minutes of exercise a day. I do forty-five to sixty. Am I overdoing it? I don't think so. I'm careful to listen to what my body is trying to tell me. If one group of body parts is sore one day, I'll work a different group the next. And I keep a constant watch on my neurological signs, my heart rate, my cholesterol levels.

Most important, I think, is a positive attitude—and I've

been blessed with a heaping helping. It was an aspect of my personality long before I had my strokes, and I've turned it up a notch since. I try to look at every situation through a rose-colored lens. For example, the very first speech I ever gave to a group of stroke patients was at the Marriott in Orlando, where I appeared at a National Stroke Association event. I spoke to a room full of people in wheelchairs and walkers and first heard the phrase *stroke survivors*. I told the survivors and the caregivers that I would always be there for them. It was the first time I considered myself lucky—because I could move, I could shave, I could drive.

There were a lot of tears in that room that day, some of them mine. You can come to after a stroke and say, "Woe is me." Or you can get busy. This was me, getting busy.

I used to think I was invincible, that life went on forever. Now that I'm older I realize, hey, it can all end one day. And it will. Today. Tomorrow. Sometime in the distant future. Count on it. Stroke didn't teach me that, but it certainly reinforced it for me. Big-time. It was an in-your-face reminder that life is finite. I've always said that life is a marathon and not a sprint, and that there is no one course we are all meant to follow. You might know where you're going one moment, and have absolutely no idea the next. Or you might know where you want to end up and have no clue how to get there. That's why I now look on each day as a precious gift. I sound like a Hallmark card, I know, but that's really how I feel. I didn't necessarily feel that way before, but I do now. The people closest to me know how much I love them. My wife, my kids, my friends and family . . . I don't miss a chance to tell them what they mean to me. Trust me, my loved ones are well-hugged, and it's because of them that I've determined to do everything in my power to ensure that I'm around for a good long while. Now I have every reason to take good care of myself.

Early on, I took my cue on diet and exercise from a woman I met at an art gallery opening in Orlando. The co-owner, Valerie Greene, was a stroke survivor and an accomplished author. I met her over dinner at my general manager's house in my early days of recovery, so a lot of the talk in the gallery was about stroke and rehabilitation. It was in this climate that a woman approached me and told me she'd had a stroke five years earlier. It was so severe they had to do brain surgery to repair some of the damage. And here she was, talking and moving without effort or ill effect. Really, you'd never know anything had ever happened to her.

I looked on and tried to imagine the bent and broken woman she described, but I got back nothing beyond radiant health and good cheer.

"My voice used to be like yours," this woman said. This was when I was still slurring some of my words. "Hang in there," she said. "It gets better."

Let me tell you, I came out of that gallery raring to go. The take-away for me was that a full recovery was within reach. I had thought my voice would never return to broadcast timbre, that I'd never cross a room with grace or aplomb.

And here was this vibrant, energetic, completely able-bodied woman to set me straight.

The more stroke patients I met, the more I started to think how the old timetables for recovery no longer applied. One of the reasons the timeline was changing, I came to realize, is because the population is changing. *We* are changing. Here we are, rewriting the literature and our own prognoses on the back of hard work and a healthier approach. It's a generational change, a new point of view. These days, more and more stroke patients are baby boomers. That's just demographics. We don't live the sedentary lifestyles of our parents and grandparents. That's just accepted fact. Look around: We're the ones who insisted forty was the new thirty. Now we're claiming sixty is the new forty. And, when we're seventy and eighty, I suspect we'll still be pretty active. We refuse to remain on the sidelines.

My father tells me that when he was a kid he knew a person who had a stroke, and that person spent the rest of her days sitting on her front porch and waving and watching the world go by. She couldn't talk. She couldn't walk. Sometimes, she couldn't even wave. She could only sit and watch. But then you have to remember that folks back then used to smoke cigarettes and drink whiskey. The only heavy lifting they did was the morning newspaper, and even that, they had one of the kids bring in for them.

I'm old enough to remember when jogging was new. It used to be that when you saw someone running around the block you assumed another someone was chasing them. It was a big leap forward from those "exercise belts" our parents and grandparents used to wear, when working out was something you had done to you instead of something you went out and did for yourself. Now we run and jump and ski and hike and bike and step and spin and break a sweat at every opportunity, so it's no wonder today's stroke patient is making greater gains than ever before. We're working at it, hard. We won't be denied. And we won't let a physical therapy manual tell us when we're done healing.

We decide when we're done. Plain and simple.

Helping us along are the researchers who continue to develop new and better medications designed to speed recovery and reduce the risk of subsequent stroke. I take Coumadin, a blood thinner, to prevent the clotting in my brain that nearly killed me. I might be on it for the rest of my life, but it's a small price to pay for the peace of mind it provides. Had I been on it in November 2005, I would have likely escaped my ordeal.

I take a drug called Primidone, to reduce the shaking I still experience in my right hand, which could certainly wreak havoc on my golf game, if my golf game was worth wreaking havoc upon. Even with the Primidone I sometimes get the shakes, but they're nothing like when I first started rehab, and nothing I can't live with from here on in. Most people don't even see that my hand is shaking, that's how subtle it is.

Like a lot of people my age, I take Lipitor for my cholesterol, which was never really sky-high but just beyond the normal range. Now, though, I need to be double-sure to keep my cholesterol in check. Here again, it's not such a big deal, and there's a great benefit to my health in general. It's helped me a bunch. I've even met doctors who take it to keep their own levels in check, before their cholesterol has a chance to climb.

I also take medication for my high blood pressure, but I'm hoping to discontinue this as soon as possible. Already, as I move further and further into exercise and lose more weight, my blood pressure has become less and less of an issue. I also take vitamins every day: C, B$_{12}$, and a multivitamin.

I used to take a lot of risks in front of the network news cameras, but nowadays I'm all about lowering risk. That's another one of my mantras: *reduce risk*. I see people who are heavy and I think, That's not good. I see people who smoke and I think, That's not good. I see people who drink too much coffee and I think, That's not good. I see people who don't exercise and I think, That's not good. Eating healthy, eating right, eating *less*...these are things we can't stress enough, as we look to reduce the risk of stroke. When you're younger, you don't think about all the things you're doing wrong. Your body is still able to compensate. You can absorb your mistakes and transgressions. But when you're older, and when someone points out to you what you could be doing to take better care of yourself, you should start listening, because your body isn't able to compensate the way it used to. The odds that had once been long in your favor are now stacked against you.

One of the messages I share with stroke survivors around the country is how important it is not to let stroke define who you are. I want people to know there's hope out there, that there are people just like them, going through the same motions, making positive strides, but at the same time they shouldn't think the rest of their lives will be all about stroke.

F. Scott Fitzgerald once wrote that there are no second acts. I disagree. My first act, at CBS, brought me into direct contact with politicians, athletes, movie stars, musicians, authors, and business leaders, and allowed me to offer my unique worldview to millions of television viewers. My second act is just beginning, but I think it might be bigger than the first. Now it's all about reaching people, making a positive difference, and spreading the all-important message that the risk of stroke can be minimized and that stroke doesn't define who you are, just as it cannot define what you will become. My father also tells me that if I can inspire just one person to get off the couch and change his or her lifestyle and prevent just one stroke, I will have done my job.

I fully expect to spend the rest of my "second act" speaking out on behalf of stroke survivors, but it's not just about stroke. It's about overcoming any and all obstacles. Stroke. Heart attack. Cancer. It's about breaking barriers and charting new territory. If someone says you can't do something, tell yourself you can. If someone sets limits on what you might achieve, look past them. If someone says you don't have a shot, take one anyway.

Denise gave me a book on golfing for my birthday. Before my strokes, golf was becoming a favorite pastime. Now, with the help of the constraint therapy program and some of the other physical therapy work I've been doing to recapture strength and dexterity in my right hand, I'm trying to get my game back. It's still not back to where it was. It'll get there, I'm sure. Eventually. (There's that word again.)

The title of the book was *These Guys Are Good*, and in one of the chapters, by Melanie Hauser, I found a quote that's stayed with me: "It's not what you accomplish in life, it's what you overcome."

I read that and thought, That about covers it.

Think about it: Everybody's got something to overcome. Sooner or later, everyone gets dealt a lousy hand. For me, lately, it's stroke. Someday soon, it will be something else. And whatever it is, I will have the strength and resolve and focus to get through it. I will press on. If you've read this far, chances are it's lately been about stroke for you as well. Someday soon, it will be something else. And whatever it is, I hope and pray that you too will have the strength and resolve and focus to get through it, and that your second act will be as big and bold and brave as your first.

ADDITIONAL RESOURCES

There are two wonderful organizations that every stroke patient and caregiver should know about. The American Stroke Association, a division of the American Heart Association, is located in Dallas, Texas, and offers a wealth of information on stroke prevention and treatment. The National Stroke Association, located in Centennial, Colorado, offers additional information. Contact and Web site information for each organization is listed below.

American Stroke Association
A Division of the American Heart Association
7272 Greenville Avenue
Dallas, TX 75231

1-888-4-STROKE
www.strokeassociation.org

National Stroke Association
9707 E. Easter Lane
Centennial, CO 80112
1-800-STROKES
www.stroke.org

ACKNOWLEDGMENTS

There are a number of people, organizations, and institutions I wish to thank, for all of their help, expertise, and encouragement. Many of them, I've been able to mention previously in these pages; many more, I have not. In no particular order, they are...

Gotham Books, especially Bill Shinker, Lauren Marino, and Brianne Ramagosa, for giving me the chance to share my experience and perspective with other stroke survivors... Orlando Regional Rehabilitation Institute... the Brain Injury Recovery Center, and all the rehab specialists there, including Courtney Muller, Lisa Ballot, and Melanie Ferraro, who always made me laugh through the healing... Sand Lake and Lucerne Hospitals, and their wonderful staffs... The

William Morris Agency, particularly Jim Griffin, my agent, whose kind words meant so much to me and who has been by my side from the beginning...Jim brought me to literary agent Mel Berger, the best there is, and a soothing, calming presence...Mel put me together with Dan Paisner, a great writer, an even better person...

Grada Fischer, the head of the Fischer Ross Group, who helped bring me back and has become a great friend...Dr. Max Medary, Dr. Nicholas Bagnoli, and Dr. John Hirt...all the kind people at WKMG, including Jacqueline London, Allison McGinley, and Darren Caudle, who put together *A Miracle of Love*...CBS News and the CBS television network, where I worked for fifteen years...*The Early Show* family: Julie Chen, Hannah Storm, René Syler, and Dave Price...it was a pleasure to be interviewed by my friend, Harry Smith, in a piece produced by producer par excellence Scott Fraser and championed by my dear friend Cathy Black...the National Stroke Association...Diane Mulligan-Fairfield, who put me on the cover of *StrokeSmart* magazine and has become a friend...we've been on many adventures together...Hip Hop Stroke, which teaches kids lifelong healthy habits and uses kids to educate their families about stroke...National Stroke Association CEO James Baranski...the American Heart Association and the American Stroke Association, and its CEO, Cass Wheeler...Pamela Garmon-Johnson, Jeff Walters, and Toiya Honore...Larry Bloustein, who does great things for the American Heart

Association and the American Stroke Association and is also a dear friend...

"The Power to End Stroke" campaign, which helps to spread the word about preventing strokes...James Taylor, of Taylor's Fitness Club—we do have fun working out...Tammy Bennett and the Longwood Preventive Medicine Group, for acupuncture and laser treatments...Central Florida Hyperbaric... Tuscawilla Country Club and Mike Gardner...Orlando Regional Healthcare, and Tracey Briggs and Sabrina Williams...my cousin David, who called every single day and whom I love very much...Dorothy Holtgrefe, my good friend, who read early drafts of this book and helped me decide what was in and what was out...the people of Orlando who've been so kind to me and my family...and, most of all, the community of stroke survivors and their caregivers...there is hope...M.M.